ne
laYground
otting shed

inic Murphy is a journalist and
Guardian's former gardening editor

the Playground Potting shed

A foolproof guide to gardening with children

Dominic Murphy

guardianbooks

Published by Guardian Books 2010

2 4 6 8 10 9 7 5 3 1

First published in Great Britain in 2008 by
Guardian Books
Kings Place, 90 York Way
London N1 9GU

www.guardianbooks.co.uk

A CIP catalogue record for this book is available from the British Library

ISBN 978-0-85265-209-1

Designed and set by www.carrstudios.co.uk
Printed and bound in Great Britain by CPI Bookmarque Ltd, Croydon, Surrey

For Hannah, Martha and Dora

Acknowledgments

This book was written over a relatively short but intense period, where weekends and evenings became a non-stop working pattern, leaving little time for family life. A huge amount of love and thanks, then, must go to Hannah, Martha and Dora for their tolerance and support.

A big thank you, also, to all the children in the gardening club at our local school, whose efforts have not only produced a garden we can all be proud of, but are the basis for this book and will hopefully be inspiration for others. I hope they have enjoyed the planting and growing as much as me.

Finally, thank you to my publisher, editor and fellow gardener Lisa Darnell, whose enthusiastic backing made the book possible. Good luck with the new allotment.

contents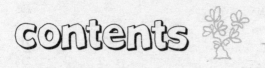

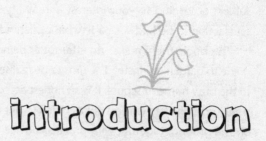

introduction

The idea behind this book, pure and simple, is to get more young people gardening - whether at home or at school, with their parents, teachers or both. It draws on my experience of running the gardening club at my local primary school in Dorset, and describes how, starting with a battered polytunnel and two patches of hopeless, waterlogged clay, we built up a beautiful, productive garden that supplied the school kitchen with vegetables and salad.

Despite the emergence of youthful presenters on TV gardening shows and attempts to show real solutions to normal-sized plots, gardening still struggles to connect with many people, notably children and young families. The impression lingers that gardening is for those with time on their hands, acres of space and, sometimes, money to pay for hired help. There is a perception, also, that horticulture takes years to master, requiring an understanding of Latin before you can find your way around plant names, and ideally a smattering of chemistry, biology and physics, too.

But no one should be put off gardening, no matter how large or small the available outside space. Yes, gardeners with 40 years' experience are still learning things, and you can dig deeper into the subject according to your interest and ability, but there is much satisfaction to be had with a few basics behind you.

This book, then, makes no attempt at being a comprehensive guide to gardening. Instead, it aims to be realistic, whether applied to the busy home or school. It is an honest account of the setbacks, small triumphs and corners cut as I tried to get the gardening club off the ground, together with practical advice that might make a garden a success.

It is both a beginners' guide, one that makes no assumptions about your horticultural skills, and a useful tool for the gardener with more experience, stripping down a huge subject to a blueprint that really works. I hope, therefore, it will prove useful for any teacher or parent who wants to do something similar in their school, or who is looking to get their children digging at home.

The practicalities of running a school garden are not always clear. You can find plenty of advice in books and on the internet about growing plants, but even the information geared towards schoolchildren seldom tackles one of the most important issues: how do you grow things to fit the academic year? A constant theme throughout the book, therefore, is timing your garden so that harvest and flowering do not happen in the holidays, when no one is there to enjoy them.

The book is divided into two parts, the first of which describes how our small group of four- to 11-year-olds made the garden from humble beginnings. In some ways, our school has a lot in common with others: little time, fewer resources. In other ways, we are lucky, having a large area of outside space that we can use. Even so, the book is designed to be relevant to a variety of gardens, however big or small – from those that consist of no more than a yard to those that take up the corner of a playing field.

In the second part of the book, I have put together a plan of how a gardening club could work through the school year. Although we started our club in the summer term, the plan in the book runs from the end of spring half term (late February/early March) to the end of autumn half term (late October). For each week during this period, I have suggested a main gardening activity, mostly based around sowing or planting. As the season progresses, and there is more to do in the garden, you might not want to sow new seeds each week but instead concentrate on what is already growing. But if there is an appetite to do more, there are plenty of other seasonal ideas in the book.

I worked with schoolchildren of primary age, but the book is just as relevant to older children. A broad bean or potato is exactly the same thing, whether grown by a six-year-old or a teenager. Neither should it be thought of as a book that is just for schools – there is nothing to stop parents, carers and their children doing at home what we achieved in term time.

At our school, the main emphasis is on growing food, and this is reflected in the book. The timing could not be more significant. Sales of vegetable seeds now outstrip those of ornamentals and there is a huge drive – from government, through national bodies such as the Royal Horticultural Society, to local groups – to encourage gardening among young people. This is not only so that children can connect more with their environment, but so that they can better understand where their dinner comes from. However, I am aware that some readers might be more interested in other aspects of gardening, such as creating a wildlife area, a pond or herbaceous border, so there are plenty of ideas for non vegetable growers, too.

To encourage a love of plants and growing things, together with some understanding of the natural world, can surely be no bad thing. But in the book I go a stage further, and gardening sustainably and in an environmentally friendly way are strong themes that run through its pages. Gardens should not only be for pleasure and growing food – they are now recognised as important habitats for wildlife and repositories of organic waste.

At our school gardening club, a major frustration is the lack of time – we only meet once a week, on Tuesday lunchtimes. As a result, we have rotas for those jobs that need doing in the interim, such as watering, and I keep my fingers crossed that the children will not forget. But a school garden, and the wealth of opportunity it provides for learning, could be much more integrated into the teaching day. Throughout the book, therefore, there are suggestions for outdoor-related activities and projects that could bring gardening into the classroom and the curriculum.

The plants I have concentrated on are simple to grow, and the varieties are tried and tested. After all, why make the process more difficult than it needs to be? Why risk disappointment when success is so easy to achieve? Read on, and you'll see what I mean.

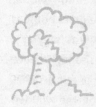

Part One

from tiny acorns

Headquarters

With no one to run it, the gardening club at my children's school had fallen by the wayside. It is probably the sign of a good school when it has, as ours does, so many clubs and out-of-classroom activities that it is difficult to keep up with what's going on. But the more extra-curricular activities you provide, the more volunteers you need to keep them going, which is where the problem begins.

At the time I took over, the gardening club occupied one corner of a generous playing field that surrounds the school on all four sides. Our territory consisted of two small patches of earth dug out of the turf, with a polytunnel as our headquarters.

The polytunnel was, and still is, both our nursery and tool shed. A row of paving slabs runs down the middle with, at one end, two metal bookcases containing hand tools and seed trays. I keep meaning to find a home for these elsewhere, to free up more planting space, but at the moment it's yet another entry in my to-do list.

At the other end of the polytunnel are some small tables of the type you find in primary school classrooms, which here double as potting benches. Apparently there's a school in Suffolk with a greenhouse climate-controlled by computers. The greenhouse is also, naturally, equipped with proper benches (known as 'staging'). We tend to be more improvisational, lacking the money to have it any other way, or the time to sort it out. On top of our benches are aluminium cooking trays. These keep water off the wooden table tops and also act as a water reservoir for pots and seed trays. There are two ways of controlling the temperature inside: door open and door shut.

But we get by. We might lack fancy equipment but we're not sloppy. One of the children's favourite activities, I have found, is tidying the polytunnel. So beneath the benches is our resource of dozens of neatly stacked, mostly plastic, pots that quickly get used up as we get busier in late spring and early summer.

The polytunnel, though, has seen better days. The doors are polythene flaps kept in place by decaying slats of wood. Grab one of them in the wrong place and you risk a nasty splinter. On very wet days, working under the plastic shell, you can never stay entirely dry. The polythene has lots of little holes in it, the result of small people trying to manoeuvre long-handled tools in a confined space.

Still, it keeps the worst of the weather out and it is here, providing the group is not too big, that we can work when it's raining or too cold outdoors. That way, the children keep dry and their clothes stay clean (in theory). Getting to the polytunnel involves a walk over boggy grass from the school building. It still amazes me what a mess this short distance can make of shoes, tights or trousers.

Despite its cosmetic shortcomings, the polytunnel has proved invaluable for the club and is a real treat for me. When I started teaching at the school, I had never had the luxury of a space to garden indoors. It extends the gardening year both sides of the growing season, and provides more options for activities in early spring and autumn, as well as giving plants a head start so they are performing or cropping before the summer holiday. I do actually own a greenhouse that I scavenged from a couple who didn't want it in their new home, but at the time I began the gardening club it lay in bits outside, waiting for me to find time to put it back together. Another entry on my to-do list.

If you have room outdoors, and can raise the money, I would always recommend a greenhouse or polytunnel. Ideally, it should be sited in a sheltered position, away from frost and wind. It should not be under branches nor too close to hedges, the idea being to maximise the light it receives all year round. Traditionally, the ridge of a greenhouse runs from east to west so that one side always gets the sun.

A greenhouse or polytunnel is the ideal scenario, but needs cash and space. If either is in short supply, you could always consider a mini greenhouse, which typically sits against a wall, is around 50cm wide and is very cheap (around £25). This, at its most basic, is a set of shelves with a plastic cover which will hold enough seedlings to kick start a good-sized veg patch. The leading chef and garden enthusiast Rose Gray, one half of the pair behind the River Café restaurant, grows salad and herbs in two cheap mini greenhouses on her roof terrace. If it's good enough for her ...

The lessons begin

Our first session was at the beginning of the summer term, in late April. The timing was by accident rather than design. The school had been casting around for someone to take over the gardening club since the beginning of the year, but it was only a week or so before we started that I decided to give it a go.

In terms of planning, it was a case of the blind leading the willing. I had not thought through what the gardening club would entail, or how we would fill our weekly sessions through the term. What if the children ignored me? Would there be discipline problems? How would I keep them entertained? I had had good teachers and bad ones when I was at school, the former being truly exceptional people. It was not a characteristic I recognised in myself.

And the timing? Well, this could have been better: while not a disaster (we could still plant things to harvest before the end of term) it was far from ideal. Our sessions only lasted for an hour, each Tuesday lunchtime, and if the children were to get any satisfaction in terms of reaping what they had sown, we would have to cram a lot into our first two weeks.

The result was that I arrived that first week with enough seeds to populate several allotments, even though we had only two little areas of open ground, each around 3m by 3m. I suppose I panicked. I was not sure how many children would turn up or how the session would work out and I squirmed at the thought of anyone getting bored. An excess of seeds would surely keep everyone busy. And besides, time was not on our side. It was sow plenty now, or forget gardening club for this term.

Thankfully, to give gardening club some semblance of an official activity, and to lend some moral support, I had a member of staff to help me. On that first day, Mrs T arrived with a list of children whose parents had signed them up for the session, and I figured she could also be my enforcer should things get out of hand. Just her presence, I felt, gave the sessions some kind of authority. She was a teacher, after all: she drank her coffee in that hallowed place called the staff room, presided over proper lessons and gave permission to go to the loo. The children would no doubt respect this. It certainly gave me more confidence in what I was doing.

Mrs T was also there to be my minder. To be allowed to work with children, you need to pass two checks made with the police and other relevant bodies. One of these is called list 99, which the school can check immediately once they have your date of birth. The other is with the CRB or Criminal Records Bureau, and takes longer to come through. Again, the school can sort this out for you, but while this is being processed, you must always be in the line of sight of a member of staff.

Mrs T stayed for the whole of the term, meaning that on busy days we could divide the group into two. By the time she left gardening club because of other staff commitments, I had got into my stride and begun to know many of the children. Having established ourselves as a real club, the idea of running it on my own was now much less daunting.

Sowing seeds

That first day, more children turned up than were on the register, meaning there were about 15 of us. I say 'about' because a couple of children drifted off halfway through, while some more arrived to see what was going on. It would always prove to be like this: children on their lunchtime break would notice something was afoot in the corner of the playing field and wander over to see what was happening. Some would stay and watch, others would get stuck in, making any notion of a gardening club 'membership' tenuous. We soon ditched the register altogether.

All ages in the school, from four- to eleven-year-olds, were represented. Although I was neither for nor against mixing abilities, it was a recipe for chaos. The smaller children, some of who were still in shock to be away from their parents for the whole day, needed constant attention if they were to get much from the session. Sometimes an older girl could be persuaded to help out but soon they would realise that this was not where the real action was and would appear at my side a few minutes later. Meanwhile, the couple of four-year-olds that had been left in her charge would now be chucking mud at each other.

I could barely keep tabs on numbers, and was hopeless with names, so it was handy that both my daughters turned up for this first session and would become regulars: if in doubt, I could quietly ask them to remind me of someone's name.

There was also the issue of what to call me. Was it going to be Dominic or Mr Murphy? All the adults at the school were known as Mr, Mrs or Miss, so perhaps I should uphold a system that was designed to instil respect among the students. How would it reflect on me if I were called Dominic – the simple gardener who did not warrant a formal title like other grown-ups? Were primary-aged children cynical enough to think that this was a lame attempt to be cool? I agonised over this – oh, for about one second – before deciding that I would introduce myself to the children as Dominic.

We gathered round in a group outside the polytunnel and I asked all the children to introduce themselves. I already knew some of them – Annie, Sasha and Esme – so I could concentrate on the unfamiliar faces. Then to work. It was a bright, clear day and not too hot, so it was perfect for working outside. I briefly demonstrated filling a pot with compost and sowing a seed, then split the group in half and let the children get stuck in.

At first we concentrated on large, easy-to-handle seeds that I thought would germinate quickly and guarantee results that term.

Sunflowers could be taken home when large enough, while nasturtiums would be blooming by July. And all being well, broad beans would crop before we broke up for the holidays. Broad beans are tough and don't actually need warmth to germinate while some varieties can be sown outside in winter, but I guessed that being sheltered under plastic would help them along.

I walked around handing out individual seeds like precious rations, getting the children to sow them individually in smaller pots or two in larger, 10cm versions. Not all the seeds we sowed that day were straightforward, including the tobacco plant (nicotiana) and tomatoes. Both of these plants have fiddly seed and their sowing needs close supervision, otherwise you will be hard-pressed to know what has been sown where, and how thickly, thinly or deep. On page 67, I have listed some general dos and don'ts about sowing but there's one over riding tip when working with children. With any small seed, never, ever, give a child the packet, unless you have sufficiently lightning reactions to grab it from them before they accidentally pour the contents on the floor.

Later in this book, and with hindsight, I suggest sowing these seeds at different times. There are two important points. First, there is no single perfect time in the gardening calendar for sowing a particular plant: you have to be flexible depending on the weather and whereabouts in the country you live. Secondly, even if you have left your gardening until the summer term, it is still not too late to begin.

We got through a disproportionate amount of seed that first day, a substantial amount of it ending up anywhere other than where it was supposed to be. At the end of the hour, however, some pots were inside, neatly labelled and on the polytunnel 'staging'. Unfortunately, there were more pots strewn around on the grass outside the polytunnel, some filled up, others half empty or on their sides. This did not look like a textbook seed-sowing session – if such a thing exists – but I sensed the children had enjoyed themselves. Some plants would surely grow from these wobbly beginnings, and that's all that counts.

But I wanted to be sure. An advantage with larger seed is that you can poke around in the pot to check that there is something in there, so after the children had gone back for afternoon assembly, I went through some of the pots outside the polytunnel, finding the seed or putting in a new one where it was needed. As for the tobacco plants and tomatoes, I sowed a tray of each myself. I didn't think of this as cheating: more of an insurance policy.

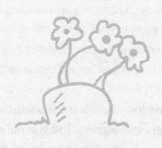

How to water

When I took over the gardening club, without a strategy and with no professional experience of working with children, I wondered how I would best keep their attention. I needn't have worried. 'Just give them a watering can and you're off,' said one teacher friend who had done some gardening with children.

It didn't take long to see what she meant. For children, watering things must be up there with ice cream and chocolate in terms of enjoyment. And like ice cream and chocolate, they don't know when they have had enough.

At the end of our first session, after Mrs T took the younger children back into school, I suggested to the others that the seeds should have a drink before we wrapped up. I might as well have organised a fight. I had barely finished speaking before the squabbles began over our three watering cans, with everyone insisting on a go before going back into school. And Annie helpfully suggested the hose. A compromise was reached with two or three children taking it in turns to hold on to a can at the same time, while I hovered over them, making sure that none of the pots or trays got too much water. We must have looked ridiculous, but no one seemed to care.

Since then, I have lost count of the seedlings we have lost in the polytunnel through overwatering. This was not down to foul play – just too much love. I would go on and on at the children about keeping seed compost damp, not soaked, but try stopping a child from watering when they've just watched their classmate do it. A child with a watering can is like a dog with a bone – no amount of persuasion will get them to give it up.

Little has changed since then: any seeds that do germinate are sometimes killed off by the watering can. This is compounded by the fact that the roses (not the plant kind, but the shower-like widget on the end of the can that ensures the water comes out as fine spray) keep on disappearing. At the time, I blamed the combined class of Reception and Year One, who had started to build a rival garden in their fenced-off playground (which I secretly hoped would not upstage our efforts), but I had no proof. Anyway, I was hardly going to start a row over a plastic widget.

But having no rose just made things worse. Seedlings that were supposed to get a sprinkle of water would regularly get drowned by a tidal wave.

One solution I have tried is to sit the seed trays in larger trays containing a bit of water, but often these would mysteriously fill up during the week between gardening club meeting, and the compost would be so soaked it looked like mushroom soup. Seeds would rot and not germinate, or germinate and then rot.

In the cooler weather of spring and autumn terms, when the compost doesn't require much watering to keep it damp, I have found the best solution is to water the seed trays myself, and risk the whole project by banning the children from their favourite thing. Watering, when you think about it, is partly common sense: when the greenhouse/polytunnel or windowledge is very warm, water more. In cooler months, water less.

During that summer term, however, the pots and trays needed to be kept moist, so I set up a rota of the older children, who would work in pairs, to cover the four days of the school week either side of gardening club. On Tuesdays, the younger ones could step in, under close supervision.

As time went on, I found that containers were the solution to the gardening club's obsession with watering. Even on wet days, when potted plants don't look thirsty, no harm will be done giving them a good drink – providing the container is well drained. Remember, entreat the children not to slosh the water in so it displaces the plants – perhaps give them a rose if you can find one. And while they are doing this, you have time to concentrate on – or perhaps even defend – your seed trays.

soil: the basics

Understand your soil, its strengths and its weaknesses, and you have overcome the biggest hurdle in running a successful school garden. Once you have the measure of the earth you are planting into you will know how to get the best from it and, where necessary, help it to improve. Is the soil is alkaline or acidic? And how does it drain? There are surely parallels here with a child's academic and emotional development.

If you are starting from scratch, say making raised beds where nothing existed before (*see page 50*) or using large containers that need filling, you might have to buy in topsoil. Topsoil – you've guessed – is the uppermost and best quality layer of soil of the garden and should be at least 20cm deep.

At our school, we were lucky when we made our raised beds because one of the parents, a groundworks contractor, gave us the earth we needed to fill them – all six tonnes of it. If you end up having to buy your earth – and there are plenty of ads for suppliers in the local paper – make sure it is 'screened', meaning it should be free of lumps of rock and plant debris.

Soil make-up

All soils consist of mineral particles, water, air and organic matter. The latter refers to the remains of plants and animals and micro-organisms. Though it plays an important part in the soil, organic matter only accounts for around five per cent of the total.

Soils tend to be identified according to the mineral particles in them, and are usually described as either sandy, silty or clay. Clay is what's known as a 'heavy' soil while sand is a 'light' soil. Think of them at opposite ends of a spectrum, with most garden soils somewhere in between, containing varying proportions of clay and sand.

A sandy soil does not hold water well. This means it has good drainage, but nutrients soon leach out of it and it is prone to erosion. However, being a light soil, it is easy to work and warms up quickly, meaning it has the potential for early sowing of crops. It is popular among market gardeners because they are able to extend their growing season; any nutrient deficiencies are balanced out by feeding, any lack of water by irrigation.

Clay soils hold water well and are potentially more fertile than sandy soils because they are better able to hold certain nutrients. They are slow to heat up at the beginning of the year and can have problems with drainage, as the children and I know all too well from our experiences at school. In summer, they can bake rock-hard and crack, like those pictures you see of empty reservoirs in a drought.

A silty soil is somewhere in between clay and sand: it retains moisture well, but drains better than clay.

Soil-wise, the holy grail for gardeners is what they call 'loam', which is probably not the same loam a geologist would recognise and which seems to have varying definitions depending on who you talk to. Loam, from a gardener's perspective, is having your cake and eating it – it combines the best elements of clay and sandy soils, being fertile, rich in organic matter and able to hold moisture, yet at the same time it is easily worked and not liable to become waterlogged.

Two other types of soil are chalk and peat. Chalk is easily identified by flecks of white in the earth, and you'll often find a very thin layer of topsoil in a chalky area. Peat – black, moist – is great on water retention but low on nutrients.

The good news is that structure and fertility in most soils can be changed and improved by the addition of organic material such as compost. (Manure, if you can get it, is great for improving the structure of soil, but should be used carefully.) The exception is peat. Peat will vary depending on where you live (the Fenland peats in East Anglia are fertile and moisture-retentive), but they are acid soils and it is best to grow plants suited to these conditions, such as rhododendrons, ferns and heathers. Some vegetables and fruit that tolerate acid soils are potatoes, fennel and raspberries.

The acid test

The acidity or alkalinity of a soil is measured by the pH scale running from 0 (acid) to 14 (alkaline). Although many plants tolerate a wide range of pH levels, a slightly acidic soil (pH6.5, where neutral is pH7) is seen as the optimum soil for the gardener. A soil that is too acid or too alkaline affects the availability of nutrients. A soil that is too acid is relatively easy to correct under an organic regime using lime – the amount you need will depend on whether the soil is clay or sand – or wood ash in small amounts. Correcting a soil that is too alkaline is more difficult – seaweed sprays help, and working in organic matter, too – although it's more common to find soil that's too acidic than soil that is too alkaline.

The pH of a soil has nothing to do with whether it is clay or sand. Peat makes acidic soil, and is again the odd one out because it will not respond to liming.

Manure

Manure is hard to get hold of if you live in a town or city: it's not like London streets are awash with the stuff, as they were in Victorian times when carriages and carts were one of the main ways to get around. And if you are able to get hold of manure, will it have any residues of antibiotics, say, that have been used to treat the animals it has come from? This is becoming more of an issue with gardeners who, if not holding all the paperwork to say they are organic, nevertheless try to run their garden on organic principles.

At gardening club, one of the girls whose mum is a farmer brought in bags of some nicely rotted manure for us to use, and it was hardly appropriate for me to quiz her about the quality of her muck. It went on to the ground along with bagged compost from the garden centre.

If you do get manure, make sure it is well rotted before using it – underneath the surface, it will be friable like good compost. Don't use fresh manure on the garden because it will burn tender plant growth and take nitrogen out of the soil while it rots down. If it is not ready to go on the garden you can either:

1) put it on the compost heap, where it will help speed up the composting process and give you a wonderful conditioner for your soil in months to come, or

2) leave it in a corner to rot down, in which case you should cover it with old compost bags or plastic to stop nutrients leaching out of it in the rain.

If manure is used too much on the same part of the garden, the soil can become too acidic. Use it once every two or three years.

What are your alternatives? Your garden centre might sell pre-bagged organic manure and there are websites that claim to sell it. Or you could do what we are trying to do at gardening club and produce lots of homemade compost – perhaps, I admit, topping it up every now and then with the bought-in variety.

The term continues

Over the following weeks we sowed pumpkins, courgettes and lettuces in the polytunnel while, outdoors, potatoes went into one of our small patches of earth. (*See Part Two for a week-by-week guide to planting these vegetables.*)

How did we pay for it all? Well, a few seeds in plastic trays and pots hardly requires a second mortgage. We were lucky in that we already had some tools, the polytunnel and enough pots to decorate an ocean liner. Our biggest expense was general purpose compost for potting, for which the school reimbursed me with the proviso that I didn't get carried away. The cost of seeds on a plot the size of ours is affordable, and in many cases I used surplus from my own garden.

The potatoes we put in were a gamble: salad spuds that I hoped would crop before the end of term. The pumpkins and the courgettes would become small seedlings in a few weeks, and although we wouldn't plant them at school (they wouldn't be ready before the summer holidays) the children could take them home at the Whitsun half term. I have no idea whether any of the courgettes survived to adulthood, but I saved a couple for myself – my children were in the gardening club after all, so why not? – and they did well planted in the compost heap at home. I know that at least one pumpkin made it through to harvest, because one of the dads thanked me for it the following term. 'Didn't eat any, mind,' he said. 'Far too small.'

Salad leaves are not famed for their popularity with children, yet they would become one of the key features of our school garden.

29

They mature fast, so are rewarding to grow and can be dotted around in any gaps that appear among flowers or other vegetables.

Another good reason to grow plenty of salad is that you can guarantee it is chemical free. Unlike root vegetables that are grown underground and get peeled before eating, pesticides sprayed on to salad leaves go directly on the bits you are eating. Commercially grown salad can be sprayed with up to 11 pesticides, more than any other crop.

Call me deluded, but I think the argument has been won about gardening on environmentally friendly grounds. It is not difficult: you just have to lower your expectations about results, which makes it even more exciting when you get a bumper crop of veg or fabulous flowering plants. It's about eating veg that may have already been nibbled by insects, and regarding disappointments as learning opportunities rather than failures.

Many organic gardeners claim that a green regime can produce similar yields and quality to a non-organic approach. Many also say that organic fruit and vegetables taste better, too. But to get first-class yields and produce from gardens run on such principles is much more labour-intensive, and plenty of time is not what we have at gardening club. So while we subscribe to green ideas, we have to be realistic about what comes out at the end.

At school, we talk periodically about how to make things grow better and ways to ward off pests. This is usually while we are doing some other activity – I don't think the children would put up with lecturing or more classroom-style sessions. Besides, we don't have anywhere to sit.

I am careful not to mention 'organic' too much. Ruby's mum, for example, is a dairy farmer and hates the idea of organics because of the paperwork it generates; her objection is bureaucratic rather ideological.

Yet despite the number of column inches devoted to growing with nature in mind, and the current fashion for all things green, many gardeners still do not think the same way. According to a survey in the run-up to the 2007 Chelsea Flower Show, nearly half the nation's gardeners still use pellets, powders and all manner of chemical nasties, prominently displayed by most garden centres like any other commodity. It is worth remembering that some easily available pesticides have been linked to serious illnesses, while manufacturing nitrogen-based fertilisers produces disproportionate amounts of CO_2.

When you look at the carnage created by slugs and snails, especially after a wet summer like 2007, you can see why it's so tempting to nuke the lot of them, especially when many pellets claim they are harmless to pets and children. But what is not so clear is what happens to a creature that eats the poisoned slug or snail.

Some chemical treatments are still permitted for the organic gardener but for help fighting pests, fertilising and still staying green, it's best to look up some the specialist websites such as www.organiccatalog.com and www.greengardener.co.uk.

digging – or not

To dig or not to dig? For gardeners, this is the question on a scale with other big debates of modern times, such as who was the greatest, George Best or Zinedine Zidane.

Autumn has traditionally been the time to dig over your soil, clearing up after the summer, getting rid of planted debris and preparing it for planting the next year. There are several reasons to dig the soil, say its advocates. First, you are improving soil structure and aeration; secondly you are exposing pests, particularly slugs, to birds. You'll be burying annual weeds and rooting out perennial ones. And finally it is a chance to incorporate soil improvers such as compost or grit for poorly draining ground.

How deep should you dig? The depth of a spade is known as a 'spit' and this is usually sufficient for perennials, annuals and most veg, because their roots don't go too deep. But if you are preparing new ground, double digging is sometimes recommended, although most modern gardeners will tell you not to bother. This involves going down two spits deep, and often then removing some of the subsoil to replace it with organic matter.

Digging over the garden in autumn is a good way to break up soils, too. You can leave the soil in clods and just let the winter frost and weather do the rest for you. In early spring, you then dig in well-rotted organic matter, before planting.

Don't dig when it is very wet, as you'll compact the ground, which defeats the object of digging in the first place. And use a plank to stand on: this spreads your weight so there is less risk of compacting the soil. Finally, unless you are of a masochistic persuasion, don't dig when it's frosty and the earth is solid: the only benefit will be your osteopath's bank balance.

So what about leaving the soil be? The advocates of a no-dig garden argue that digging simply breaks up the complex structure of the soil. Soil is alive, a world beneath our feet that relies on a delicate balance of air, water and living organisms. By attacking this world with a crude tool that does not distinguish between weed or worm, you are harming it rather than doing it good, breaking up a complex ecosystem that you can use to your benefit. Better, say the advocates of no-dig gardening, to regularly cover the ground with home-made compost and let the worms do the work for you, pulling this goodness down into the ground. All this activity creates worm tunnels that channel air and water into the soil, while compost encourages fungi and bacteria to help plants with their rooting.

Under this regime, the only tilling of the earth that is needed is regular hoeing to keep weeds down and turn up pests, such as slugs, that live in the soil. The no-dig people see their approach as the rapier to the digger's cudgel.

While the no-dig ideal has been adopted at gardening club because it is less physically demanding, the reality is that there is room for both approaches to the garden. Digging is the best way to get a neglected, dysfunctional bit of ground up to snuff, while the no-digging philosophy is an easy way to maintain it afterwards. If you like to get stuck into your ground every autumn, as traditional veg growers have done for decades, that's for you to decide.

Seeing green

Ten easy ways to be green in the garden

1) Avoid artificial chemicals, pesticides, herbicides and fertilisers.

2) Conserve water: with the possible exception of summer 2007, water shortages now seem a perennial concern of the UK gardener. You could, then, set up water butts round the school to supplement the mains supply. There are plenty of plastic butts to choose from – try garden centres or www.crocus.co.uk, or for recycled versions www.thetankexchange.com. For something less ugly, try recycled oak barrels at www.plantstuff.com. Expect to pay £20-plus for a 100-litre tank or butt.

3) Buy local: select species and veg varieties that are grown locally, so that once they are established, they should thrive and not require extra watering (this will also make them more resistant to pests and disease). If you are in an area that has low rainfall, this might mean kissing goodbye to some thirsty stalwarts of the British garden such as dahlias and delphiniums. There are, however, plenty of plants that are happy in dry conditions. Many require free-draining soil, so that they don't end up sitting in a bog when it rains. Again, do this by digging in organic matter and, if conditions are really difficult, some horticultural grit, too. Popular and easy species that are suited to baking in the sun with little liquid refreshment include lavenders, rosemary, festuca, phormiums, cistus, and varieties of sedum and euphorbia.

4) Encourage wildlife: it's basic biology, this one. Beneficial wildlife eats bad wildlife, so the good guys get a meal while your plants live to fight another day. Some examples of good wildlife include hedgehogs (encourage them with wood piles for hibernation), slowworms (they love a hot compost heap), frogs and toads, all of which are among the best predators of slugs and snails. To battle against aphids, encourage blue tits, ladybirds, lacewings and hoverflies. Birds are easy to attract with feeders (black sunflower seeds seem by far their favourite food). Ladybirds, lacewings and hoverflies can be encouraged by planting species that attract them, for example dill and fennel (which easily seeds itself). For more details on all of the above, go to www.greengardener.co.uk.

5) Dig a pond: OK, so we haven't done this at gardening club, but it is on our wish list. Beneficial creatures such as frogs need water to breed in, and a pond will attract hundreds of useful insects, from predators (dragonflies) to pollinators – check out Pond Conservation (www.brookes.ac.uk/pondaction) for information. Obviously it should be fenced off, with a latch high enough to keep out young children. And if you don't have room for a pond, a small water feature – for example, a basin sunk into the ground – will do the job. (*See page 100 for more on ponds.*)

6) Mulch, mulch, mulch: mulch is a layer of organic or inorganic matter that you put on top of the soil and around the base of a plant. This helps to a) lock in moisture and

protect the soil from the drying effects of sun and wind and b) suppress weeds that compete for nutrients and water. Mulch can be gravel, wood bark, old grass clippings or even plastic sheeting. A mulch of well-rotted animal manure also acts as a slow-release fertiliser. When watering the ground, remember to scrape or peel back the mulch beforehand. (*See page 121 for more on mulch.*)

7) Make your own compost: as if you were not planning to do this already. It takes waste out of landfill and makes a valuable soil conditioner, too. Good conservation of water goes hand in hand with horticultural best practice. A soil rich in organic matter helps plants to thrive and holds water well. That means you should regularly add compost. (*See page 121 for more on compost.*)

8) Helpful neighbours: companion planting is where plants are combined to deter pests, attract beneficial insects and, in some cases, provide nutrients for each other. The scent of coriander, chives and chervil, for example, is believed to deter aphids, so plant them near roses, say. French marigolds (*Tagetes patula*), when in flower, are used in greenhouses to deter whitefly, while carrots are often grown next to onions and garlic to deter carrot fly. And in a rotation system, beans are planted before nutrient-hungry potatoes, because their roots fix nitrogen in the soil.

9) Use green manures: animal manure can be difficult to get hold of and may contain dormant weed seeds and sometimes unacceptable chemical residues, depending on

where it has come from. Green manure is a living mulch that is sown on to bare earth, which prevents soil erosion and the leaching of nutrients and also stops weeds moving in. Any plant can act as a green manure, but there are some that are sold specifically for the task. Typically, green manures are dug in a few weeks before you plan to plant into the ground and acts as a fertiliser, too (*see page 123 for more on green manure*).

10) Make your own plant food: this is particularly useful for plants in containers where their restricted roots limit the plant's ability to find nutrients. Comfrey is probably the best known source of home-made liquid feeds, high in potassium and nitrogen. It is easy to grow, happy in a shady corner, but is invasive, so best kept away from the main garden. Collect the leaves, pack them into a bucket with a lid, then cover in water. Keep in a corner of the garden well away from where you work because the rotting leaves stink. When rotted, dilute with water until the liquid becomes a straw colour. You can do the same thing with stinging nettles (supposed to increase a plant's resistance to disease) and borage, an easy herb with blue flowers that thrives in the sunshine. This, too, produces a concentrate high in nitrogen.

Salad days

The lettuce we planted our first summer term were the crispy Cos-type Little Gem and Webb's Wonderful. Though lettuce can be sown straight outside at this time of year, we started ours off in trays. This would give the tasty leaves some protection from slugs, but equally I did not like the look of the ground around the polytunnel. You didn't need to be a geologist to take in the unpromising nature of the clay. Save for the Tarmac car park, this corner of the school grounds seemed like the worst possible place to grow things: the soil was so bad that any prolonged bout of rain turned bare earth into a bog. Conversely, in dry, sunny periods, it baked as hard as rock.

So our first batch of lettuce did not go out into open ground until it looked large enough to survive outdoors. This was towards the end of May, when it joined the broad beans, nasturtiums and some calendula I had brought from my garden. With jobs such as transplanting salad and potting on tomatoes – and an ill-considered, doubtless boring, demonstration of pruning some of the school's roses – the first half of the summer term soon went by.

The first week after Whitsun, it rained so much we cancelled gardening club and my misgivings about the ground proved justified. Our neat little scene from a child's story book, with its rows of broad beans and lettuce, became a temporary pond. The beans pulled through (I told you they were tough), but only two lettuce survived.

How to plan a garden

If you are starting a garden from scratch it really pays to make a plan. Not only should it help you develop a harmonious outside space, but it offers huge potential for fun, learning-based activities with the students and gives them a sense of ownership of the garden.

Start by assessing your site. Is it open or enclosed, mostly shady, or sunny for a good part of the day? This will determine to a large extent what you can grow. A predominantly shady garden in a narrow area between two large buildings is not the best place to raise vegetables (Jerusalem artichokes are one notable exception and will cope with partial shade). However, there are many fabulous foliage plants that thrive in the shade, such as hostas, *Fatsia japonica*, the well-behaved bamboo *Phyllostachys nigra*, ivies, Mexican orange blossom (*Choisya ternata*), and the green and white grass *Miscanthus sinensis* 'Variegatus'. Those school buildings could also provide important shelter for your plants, so you might be able to put some less hardy exotics into the mix (visit www.architectural-plants.com for ideas).

Now, make a wishlist of what you want in the garden. Will there be arches, seats, fencing, maybe even a pond? Will there be raised beds? You should think about how you will navigate the garden: ideally, it should be a garden for everyone, with wide paths easily negotiable by wheelchair (1.2m minimum width), and slopes rather than steps – although I confess we have yet to make paths in our garden.

Garden styles

There are many different styles that work well in a school garden. You'll need to decide if yours will use one sort of style or have several different 'looks' and varied planting. Ours, for example, is predominantly a kitchen garden with a wildlife area (*see page 54*). It would be good if you and the children could visit local gardens that are open to the public. Those run by the National Trust (www.nationaltrust.org.uk) are not always outrageously grand, while you can sample 'real' gardens under the National Gardens Scheme (www.ngs.org.uk).

project:

Make a plan of the garden

Take a photograph of the area you intend to develop and print it off, ideally A4 size.

Trace over this on to tracing paper, showing the key features that already exist in the space and make a few photocopies (don't forget, you can use this method to improve on an existing garden). You now have an outline on which to try out several ideas. Sketch in the features and sort of planting you would like, and see how it works together.

Our first harvest

By the second half of the Summer term, in early June, gardening club had developed a regular hardcore of members who, combined with a smattering of fair-weather friends, made for a decent turnout each week. This included Sasha, who at ten was one of the oldest in the group. Sasha had bags of ideas. When would we start a herb garden? What flowers can you eat? And I appreciated the fact that she always turned up, as well as her enthusiasm. She was the first to try the rocket we grew, when others didn't dare, and on Tuesday mornings she went round the younger children in the school, reminding them it was gardening club at lunchtime.

Sasha was desperate to harvest the potatoes, so it was a relief when towards the end of term the flowers drooped and the foliage started to die back, suggesting they were mature enough to dig up. I had been worried that they would not be ready to crop before the holidays at the end of July, but now it looked like the time had come. When I gave the go-ahead, there was a mad dash for trowels, forks and spades, as if it were some new sports day race.

As plant after plant was unearthed, there was no sign of any spuds, just the occasional lump of fetid goo, which gave a new, unpleasant meaning to the idea of mashed potato. Potatoes are used to break in difficult ground, but this clay had proved too much, refusing to let water drain away and so rotting our crop. The rot probably set in after the mid-term deluge that did for most of the lettuce. Eventually, we turned up one healthy potato. With its thin skin and white-yellow flesh it was nearly perfect and Sasha was delighted. What a pity it was only the size of a grape.

41

We had more luck with the broad beans, our other significant harvest of the term. For me, one of the main purposes of the gardening club was to encourage the children to eat more veg – or at least to try it. I had never understood the logic that if a child sees something grow they are more likely to eat it, but I was prepared to test the theory. And I knew from past experience that my youngest daughter had been persuaded to eat French beans when she picked them from our vegetable patch at home.

I knew, however, that I was stretching the point by growing broad beans. They're not exactly the easiest thing to get into a young mouth, but I had other motives for planting them. They are so hardy, I reckoned, anyone can get them to grow. In other words, at least there would be one crop to harvest this term and I would be saved the humiliation of running a gardening club that can't produce any veg. This was personal.

While it's true that anyone can grow broad beans, they are not quite problem-free, being prone to infestation with blackfly. This is one reason why many gardeners sow an early crop in autumn to harvest the following spring before the blackfly really kicks in, and don't bother with a spring sowing that is likely to get infested in the warmer months. But like so much of gardening, what applies in an ideal world has scant relevance to your own little corner. For us, planting broad beans this summer term was a case of beggars can't be choosers.

Blackfly feed on the sap of plants, causing them to eventually shrivel and die. They also breed like mad. Turn your back for a moment and a few of them have suddenly created a whole colony.

There's a big 'yuck' factor for the children but try to look closely at an infested plant, and you will see ants running around, too. Don't be lulled into thinking they are dealing with the problem. Ants feed on the honeydew secreted by the blackfly, so actually protect them from predators.

One way of preventing blackfly taking over is to encourage ladybirds in the garden, who like nothing better than aphids to feed on. You can actually buy ladybird larvae and pretty little houses in which they can overwinter along with other useful bugs and bees for the garden (try www.greengardener.co.uk or www.organic catalog.com). However, I have never seen ladybirds single-handedly stem the tide.

Another very effective remedy is to spray the blackfly on the bean plants with a weak solution of washing-up liquid, preferably a biodegradeable brand, using a plastic spray bottle you can buy at the hardware store (I actually use an old spray-cleaner bottle). I have been told variously that this blocks the creatures' pores or makes them slip off the plant, but who cares as long as it works? You have to spray regularly, however, like every day. Once a week at gardening club might be fun for whoever is in charge of the spray can, but it does not prevent the blackfly getting a foothold.

It was the week before the holidays that we picked our broad beans and true to form, many had succumbed to blackfly, the aphids so thick in places they made a lumpy film around the stems of the plants. But there were enough pods to harvest and even though some were barely recognisable, the beans inside them were untouched. It was a sweltering day – gardening clubs do not get to choose the cool, early morning for harvest – and the stickiness of insect and sweatiness of palm made for a gruesome combination. Still, some of the children rose to the challenge and began scraping off the aphids with relish (I reckoned these were the ones who also enjoy pulling the legs off spiders). Others were more squeamish, finding the whole thing too gross, and would only pick the pods that were absolutely aphid-free.

It didn't take long, though, to fill a small pan borrowed from the kitchen. We washed the beans at the outside tap and a few of us took them inside to cook them. I had an ambition – not yet shared with the children – to provide enough of something that could be part of a school dinner, but this would have to wait until next year.

Did I win any converts to broad beans? A few, I think, or maybe they were just being kind (Sasha, of course, said she loved them). Young broad beans are delicious and a totally different experience from the gnarled old bruisers you get later in the season. With that bit of added butter, perhaps the children had never had them like this before. The real success was that all but one of the children tried them. And that little girl who refused? She doesn't know what she's missing.

our first sPring

Gardening club would not reconvene until late the following February, in the first Tuesday after half term. February/early March is an ideal time to start your school garden, but remember that you will miss an important two weeks over the Easter holidays. You can use the holiday to plan what to plant for the coming season, some hardier seeds can soon go in the ground, while there is plenty to get going in a greenhouse, polytunnel or on a windowledge. There will be early potatoes to plant and you can still order good quality seeds rather than relying on leftovers in the garden centre.

Many gardeners will tell you that if you leave planting until later, then your garden will catch up. To start things too early is to risk having a glut of seedlings ready to plant out, but weather and ground that is too cold to take them – and to some extent they are right. But for a school gardening club that meets for only one hour a week, starting early is a way of spreading out all those jobs, from sowing seed to weeding and preparing the ground, that might otherwise hit you in a wave later on in the season.

Don't be influenced by the chainstore garden centres. The gardening year for them starts at Easter, whether the holiday comes at the end of March, or much later in April. This is when new stock arrives on the shelves and marketing is stepped up for the bank holiday shopper. The magazine supplements fall in line, devoting more space than usual to the subject and, of course, delighted to carry any advertising that comes their way.

That February day was clear and dry, but the patch of ground that we used for planting last summer was still sodden from the winter rain. No matter. February was too early to start things outside so I had brought with me my old stalwarts: seeds to sow inside the polytunnel.

I was pleased with the turnout. Perhaps word had spread since the summer that gardening club was a cool thing to do. Today's gathering was remarkable, however, not only for its numbers on a cold February lunchtime, but for the amount of boys present. Previously, girls were in the majority. Perhaps they were happy that this particular lunchtime's exercise extended to pulling up weeds and harvesting beans rather than battering each other in the playground. Perhaps it appealed to a nurturing instinct. Or perhaps it was more than a coincidence that both my daughters turned up every Tuesday and inevitably some of their friends would want to come, too.

My experience was that we did get some boys turning up but never that regularly: children are always dropping out or dropping in. Little Leo would often come with his big sister, and dreamy-looking Pip had a run, too. Pip's wonder at the miracle of gardening was truly rewarding – or that's how I saw it. 'Can you really eat that?' he asked me one day, marvelling at the French bean in his hand. I was touched by his naivety. Or was he trying to wind me up?

Sometimes Ben, Harry and his elder brother Matthew had put in an appearance, but their enthusiasm dwindled over time. If there was no immediate physical reward (filling a pot, digging a hole) they would drift away to something more physically stimulating – the football, cricket, war games or whatever was going on in another part of the playing field.

I always tried not to take this personally, although in moments of doubt I wondered whether our Tuesday lunchtimes might be more structured. Should we play more games? Should I turn up with props? Or was it enough that out of these chaotic hourly sessions would one day come seedlings, flowers, and even a crop of vegetables?

Today, the number of boys had been swollen by a handful of Year Fives and Sixes, the oldest children in the school. Word had got round that there was digging to be done, which was not actually the plan. It was far too wet and I had envisaged a bit of a tidy-up, catching up with old faces and learning new ones, then sowing a lot of seeds. Admittedly, there were more of us than I expected and we wouldn't all be able to squeeze into the polytunnel at once, but it was mild enough for the children to take it in turns filling pots outside, then bringing them indoors.

Most of our lessons would pan out in this way: I would have an idea of the priority for the day, but what we would end up doing would depend on numbers, so even with quite careful planning there was an element of muddling through. If we still had extra time left after the main task of the day – say, potting on tomatoes – I always made sure I had a back-up plan, such as more seeds to sow or, later in the season, a bed to prepare or weed. As the garden developed and the season got into its stride, there was always more to keep us busy than just sowing.

Today was our first meeting of the season, so my back-up was simply going to be a chat with the children, asking them what they would like to do for the rest of term and dropping hints about things that I would like to do, too.

With 12 or so children to entertain, the idea of a handful of them amusing themselves had great appeal. At the beginning of the session, one of the older boys called Charlie had suggested digging a drainage ditch at one end of our biggest mud patch. In my defence, I was distracted by other children and Charlie was very persistent, and though I don't actually remember saying 'Yes', I might have shrugged and said 'Whatever'. It would be four fewer people bugging me and maybe it would even drain some of the clay.

While the majority of the group stayed in the polytunnel, filling trays with compost and seed, Tim, Charlie, Matthew and others set to with the waterlogged clay. I suppose I had not realised just how saturated the ground had become. In a few minutes they had not only built a 'drainage' ditch at one end of our veg patch, but spattered themselves and their young spectators in mud. None of them had thought to bring wellies – no surprises there – so their shoes were caked in mud. As for their school uniforms, I just waited for the angry phone calls from their parents.

The water did actually collect in the channel dug that day, making its way from the mud patch to the lowest point of ground, but the idea was not one of the best we have had at gardening club. If I had been really prepared and planned ahead, I would have assessed my site the previous summer before any gardening activities started and begun a long course of soil improvement. (This is what they always do in gardening books, but I wonder whether life ever does imitate manuals.) Beth Chatto, who began her famous garden under similar unpromising circumstances, recommends digging in large amounts of horticultural grit, together with organic matter such as compost and well-rotted manure. And by digging she means serious excavation, down to at least the depth of two spade heads. The boys would have loved it.

But try selling soil improvement to children (apart from the handful of drainage diggers, who were, after all, not regulars). They have come expecting to grow things, so you won't get far concentrating on organic matter and improving the mud in front of you to look like … well, drier mud.

In the previous summer term, we had made a slight effort to improve the ground, taking Beth's wise words on board, but not exactly following them to the letter. We had fiddled with, rather than overhauled, our 'garden', adding as much compost as we could afford (very little), sharp sand (the poor person's equivalent of horticultural grit) and some cow manure that had been given to us by one of the parents. And because the ground was too hard for the children to dig into, it was me who did all the heavy work while an increasingly bored audience stood by. This term, the garden was marginally less of a dead loss, but there was huge room for improvement. It still turned into a mud bath whenever we had rain, and plants soldiered on rather than thriving in such miserable foundations.

Yet something positive came of the drainage ditch. For me, it was the last straw, absolute proof that it was pointless to struggle on with our contrary little bog. This was not about making the best of a bad lot – to carry on this way was gardening club suicide. The answer, if we were to make a decent fist of growing veg and flowers, was to start again and build our beds upwards.

Making raised beds

Raised beds are a no-brainer if you have rubbish soil, and now that I had seen our mud patches at their worst and had watched promising crops ruined the previous summer, it was a case of building some for ourselves or abandoning planting outdoors.

Filled with good soil and compost, raised beds are a chance to start from scratch, rather than constantly fighting to make the best of what you've got. They are a proper garden as opposed to damaged goods, the beginnings of good husbandry, a step out of the mire.

They are also a good solution if you only have a concrete backyard or small space where you want to maximise yields. They provide decent drainage, the soil warms up more quickly in the spring, and there is an extra barrier for snails and slugs to overcome. They are also perfect for wheelchair users. For children, they make a clearly defined space that they are less likely to walk on.

On the downside, they dry out quickly and any gaps between the soil and the side of the bed, or long grass around their edges, can be hiding places for pests. These, however, are very minor cons for a great deal of pros.

Raised beds do not have to be very deep, though the shallower they are, the closer they are to that rotten ground you are trying to get away from. Think deep. About 10cm is a decent minimum if you are siting them on bare earth. If you are on concrete or paving or planning them with wheelchair users in mind, the higher the better (I would allow at least 30cm). Children can help out by filling them in with soil, and/or the stones that are to be used at their base. Older children might be able to help with sawing and screwing the frames together.

Building raised beds

We made our raised beds using 10cm x 2cm green oak from a local sawmill. Green oak is newly cut timber, which means it is still full of moisture and is likely to warp, but being a hardwood it does not need treating and you should get at least a decade out of it before it rots. It is easy to find green oak that is native and from sustainable sources, so you score extra eco points here. If you are looking for a perfect solution, it is better to use untreated railway sleepers (try www.ecomerchant.co.uk) or, if you must, treated wood from a timber merchant, which will be much cheaper.

Old scaffolding boards are popular if you can get hold of them, but generally you should be wary of scrap wood. Has it been treated with creosote (you don't want that leaching into your veg), or is it covered in old leaded paint (ditto)? It was only recently that arsenic was banned from treated wood, so old timber might not be suitable either.

Width matters!

A raised bed should be no more than 1.5m wide, so that you can easily reach across it without having to stand on the soil in the middle. I found this out the hard way: our raised beds are 2m wide, and the children have to walk on them to reach the middle. Walking on bare earth not only gets mud on school shoes (I have gone on and on about bringing wellies, but at least half the group always forget), but compacts the soil and destroys its structure. If this is really necessary, have a plank handy to put on the ground and spread your weight.

Once you have the wood for the sides of the beds, it should be screwed into posts at each corner (nails will only come out). And if you understand basic physics and don't mind a rustic look, it makes sense to drive wooden pegs into the ground on the outside of the raised beds. This will help contain the soil that is pushing against the sides.

If you are putting your raised beds straight on to earth, dig this over a bit first; the worms will do the rest. We sited our raised beds on the playing fields, and all I did was to dig up the turf and turn it over (I did this out of gardening club hours because stripping turf is hard work and time-consuming, but it could be a project for willing – and strong – older children). If the beds are on top of concrete or paving, it would be good to lift or break this up beforehand. This is easier said than done, so if it is not possible, put a good layer of gravel, crocks (broken pots) or stones in the bottom (say 5cm deep) and drill drainage holes around the base of the wood.

Our four raised beds took the rest of the term and a bit of the next before they were all completed. Finding the £90 for the wood was easy enough – news of the drainage ditch fiasco had spread, and the parents who made up the Friends of the school said they would stump up the cash.

It did not take long to build the frames, either (I did this in non-gardening club time because I couldn't work out a way to incorporate it into a Tuesday lunchtime: too many dangerous tools, and too many bored onlookers). Finding something to fill them in, however, proved trickier and I wished I had asked for money for topsoil as well.

The frames for the beds were built by early March and over the following weeks, an advert in the village shop brought some small trailer-loads of home-made compost and topsoil. The earth was slowly trickling in, but it wasn't until the mid summer that all the beds were filled. One of the parents at the school, who also happened to be a groundworks contractor, came up with the necessary six tonnes of topsoil and dumped it one day in the school car park. Once more I called on the older boys, who had drifted away since the day of the drainage ditch, to help me wheelbarrow it to the beds. It took us three lunchtimes of shovelling, with two boys pushing a wheelbarrow, and they loved it. If only gardening club could be like this all the time, one of them said, as we swept up on the final day.

Planting a garden for wildlife

Why should you have a garden for wildlife? For a start, children will get a lot out of it, whether it is the grossness of turfing up a huge worm or grub or, as we had one day, the novelty of rehousing a toad. And one session was cancelled because an adder was supposed to have been seen lurking around the polytunnel. The following week, the children were more intrigued than frightened (and anyway, a dead grass snake nearby suggested it was a case of mistaken identity).

In an urban garden, it is unlikely you will have snakes as visitors, but an animal- and insect-friendly garden is still a good thing, and the reasons go far deeper than a mere sentimental affection for other living creatures.

Firstly, you will be providing a valuable habitat at a time when the pressure to develop our wild spaces is increasing. Intensive farming is still the mainstream means of cultivating food. Combine this with the added pressure on greenfield sites for housing and it's easy to understand why the countryside is on the back foot in most areas, retreating in some. Meanwhile, there are some 15 million gardens in the UK, estimated to cover about 270,000 hectares, according to the Wildlife Trusts. With that kind of reach, gardens are increasingly seen by conservation groups as an important refuge for wildlife.

Secondly, wildlife can work for you, helping to pollinate plants and keeping pests at bay. Think of it as enlightened self-interest.

But wildlife will only come knocking if you take a certain approach to your outdoor space. Being trigger-happy with the insect spray or making merry with the weedkiller won't encourage animals to move in. An immaculate section of turf that has been doused in artificial fertilisers is a desert compared to a meadow of similar size. The latter will be teeming with insects – maybe there'll be a small mammal of some sort using its cover, or even a slowworm basking in the sunshine.

Over time, a wildlife garden will find its natural balance, unfriendly wildlife being kept under control by natural predators, friendly wildlife helping plants to thrive by pollinating them and eating the pests.

Does that mean we should put up with snails, aphids and the like? To an extent, the answer is yes. Take snails, for example. They are useful, disposing of rotting vegetation and in a healthy garden, will be kept under control by birds such as thrushes. Like it or not, they are part of a finely balanced ecosystem, and while I never shy away from aggressive control of such creatures (I chuck them on to the lawn for the birds to pick them off, for example), I don't obsess about their total elimination. Most of the time. Besides, there are historical warnings about taking things to extremes. In 1950s China, Chairman Mao notoriously put sparrows on a list of pests to be exterminated in his great leap forward. The idea came back to haunt him as the policy was followed by plagues of insects that had once been controlled by the birds.

Attracting wildlife

All wildlife require four essentials: habitat, food, shelter and places to breed.

Generally speaking, it is surprisingly easy to provide all of this. If you leave small areas of your garden to go wild, you create shelter for all manner of beasts, which are in turn preyed on by other creatures.

During a spate of weed clearing in the school garden, we came across a toad that had taken up refuge in the lush cover of docks and poppies. He had to go, because our weeding had blown his cover, but we didn't want him to stray too far because toads feed on slugs. So we moved him under the nearby hedge with an old clay pot turned on its side; hopefully he will make that his home.

If you have a grassy area, allow some of the grass to grow through summer (*see An easy meadow, page 75*). This will attract insects such as butterflies, grasshoppers and moths, as well as birds and, if you have flowers, bees, too.

Heavenly hedgerows

Hedgerows are wonderful resources for wildlife. The most suitable is a mixed one, because it is more likely to attract a range of creatures. The more diverse the planting, the more varied the creatures attracted to it. Try to plant native species, which will appeal more to our indigenous animals and insects. Maybe you can throw in a tree or two as well – studies have found that any garden with a tree is better for wildlife.

Hedges provide shelter, nest sites and fruit and berries for food. A deciduous hedge will lose its leaves in autumn, giving ground cover for creatures such as beetles, and material that rots down into the soil. On the downside, they might also provide a hiding place for slugs, but better here than among your vegetables and hopefully, with that ready-made shelter and food supply, you'll get a hedgehog moving in.

If you have a hedgerow or trees, spare a thought for nesting birds and remember not to go cutting and pruning in the spring, or you'll disturb their nests and chicks.

A native hedgerow – for free

Over the past 50 years, half our hedgerows have disappeared. If you fancy planting a hedgerow in your school grounds – perhaps to divide up a part of the garden – or extending one that already exists, The Woodland Trust will give your school 30 shrubs, enough to make around 8m of hedge. Details on www.woodlandtrust.org.uk. For more information and support with planting hedgerows and trees visit BTCV (www.btcv.org.uk) and Trees for Life (www.treesforlife.org.uk).

Key native hedgerow species:

Hawthorn (*Crataegus*) Beautiful blossom, and its dense prickly interior is a haven for nesting birds. Often the main ingredient of a typical native hedgerow. Keep away from thoroughfares as its thorns are nasty.

Blackthorn (*Prunus spinosa*) Dense clusters of white flowers in spring, followed by bitter sloe fruits.

Hazel (*Corylus avellana*) Nuts for autumn sustenance and catkins in spring.

Guelder rose (*Viburnum opulus*) Maple-like deciduous leaves with good autumn colour; white flat flowers in summer popular with butterflies, followed by glossy red fruits.

Field maple (*Acer campestre*) Makes a dense hedge with leaves turning butter yellow in autumn.

Holly (*Ilex aquifolium*) A way to introduce some evergreen into your deciduous hedge. Berries in winter provide food, too. Note: to get berries on your holly you will need both male and female plants to pollinate.

Dog rose (*Rosa canina*) Wild rose with pretty single flowers and hips in autumn.

In the flower garden, insects will be searching out nectar and pollen, so try to have something in bloom from spring to autumn. Plant a range of flowering annuals, perennials and

project:

Before you plant up a wildlife garden, get students to suggest good wildlife and why you want it in your garden. Now help them to work out how to attract these animals. What are their needs? More information from www.natural-england.org.uk; www.rhs.org.uk

biennials so, in effect, you are covering all seasonal bases and likely to attract a wider range of visitors. If you plant your flowers in clumps rather than dotted around, the insects that are attracted to that particular plant will find it easier to locate. Single-flowered specimens are better for insects than modern, multi-petalled hybrids because they tend to be higher in pollen and nectar.

Plants to attract insects

Spring

Flowering currant (*Ribes sanguineum*); hawthorn; crocus; wallflower (*Erysimum cheiri*); lilac; Christmas rose (*Helleborus*); forget-me-not; prunus species (*including plum and cherry trees*).

Summer

Cornflower; rosemary; borage; California poppy; lavender; sunflower; tobacco plant (*Nicotiana*); hebe.

Late summer/autumn

Sedum spectabile; butterfly bush (*Buddleia*); honeysuckles; ivy; Michaelmas daisy (aster); *Echinacea purpurea*; French marigold (*Tagetes patula*); fennel.

Providing food for wildlife

In winter, leave seedheads on dying perennials such as sedum, Verbena bonariensis and teasels, as these provide precious food for birds when it is scarce. And think about planting species with berries, such as holly, pyracantha, cotoneaster and sorbus for the same reason.

One of the easiest ways to create a thriving habitat is to build a log pile, or simply leave some logs in a corner of the garden to decompose. Old scraps of wood are fine and will provide a home and food for a wide range of creatures from beetles and butterflies to spiders, woodlice and perhaps even a hibernating hedgehog. (If you are lucky enough to house a hedgehog in your garden, don't leave out cow's milk for it: hedgehogs are allergic to it, and will thank you much more for a small dish of cat food.)

Don't forget that gardens can grow upwards as well as horizontally – planting climbers to make use of vertical space allows wildlife to use the cover whichever way it grows. Ivy is perfect for a dark corner, and if left to get thick enough is popular with sheltering birds. Ivy flowers are one of the most important sources of winter food in the garden, so encourage it where you can.

Housing for wildlife

Think about buying nest boxes for birds. A bird box should be put up between August and February when you are least likely to disturb breeding birds, and in a sheltered spot, out of wind, rain and strong sunshine (east or north-east facing is good). Make sure the lids are secure so that squirrels and magpies cannot raid their eggs, and place them out of reach of cats, with small branches around them – enough for birds to perch, but not sufficient to take the weight of a cat. You should clean them annually in late autumn with boiling water to get rid of any mites, checking first that they are not being used as a roost. For bird boxes, see www.wildforms.co.uk.

Crop rotation

There was a good reason behind our decision to have four raised beds. On the wall above my desk is a map showing our village in 1888. As you would expect, it is very different from today and instead of a settlement of around 800 people, there are only a handful of homes, with most of the buildings grouped into three large farms. The site where the school would be built in 1975 is one of several orchards long since grubbed up, and to the north of that is the large rectory. The old kitchen garden of the rectory is now housing, but on this map it is clearly divided up into a grid of four equal squares with paths running around the outside and in between them to make a cross shape.

Victorian gardeners grew food to eat and operated a four-year rotation scheme. Every year, each of the four areas would be planted with a different botanical group of vegetables, which was then moved the following season so they only occupied the same patch of ground once every four years.

This approach prevented the build-up of pests and diseases that favour one family of plants. Its wisdom dates back to the ancients and is still followed by organic gardeners today.

Though we would eventually have four raised beds into which would go the four main families of crops, by late spring we had a glut of crops to plant out, but only soil in one-and-a-half beds. In other words, my neat plan for a rotation system would have to wait. We would put in what we could into the available garden, and avoid planting the same crop in exactly the same place next season. Gardening is so often about compromises.

But imagine for a moment that those four raised beds were up and running. How would we have planned them? The most important groups of vegetables to rotate are potatoes, brassicas (cabbages and greens), legumes (the beans family), alliums (onions) and roots such as parsnip (see below for categories). Alliums and roots are usually lumped together, along with the beet family (not as confusing as it sounds), so you end up with four groups of vegetables for your four-bed rotation scheme.

To maintain the soil in optimum condition, says Caroline Foley in her *Allotment Handbook*, potatoes should be followed by roots, then legumes, then brassicas. If you are really organised, you will manure the soil in readiness for the potatoes, which are greedy and like lots of nutrients, then add lime the following year for roots. The cycle continues with more manure for the legumes, which also fix the important nutrient nitrogen in the soil, then lime again for the brassicas. This, says Foley, will help maintain a balance in the soil, not too alkaline, not too acidic.

There are some vegetables that you need not worry about and can be slotted in where there are spaces. Many salad leaves, for example, fall into this category, as does Swiss chard, spinach and sweetcorn.

And then there are the perennial vegetables such as rhubarb, asparagus, artichoke and the spinach-like Good King Henry that will need more permanent patches in the garden.

Working out what to plant and where is an interesting exercise for children, though we were hamstrung at first with only one-and-a-bit beds. Still, they got the point of avoiding the same thing in the same place, year after year. They can hone the idea, as I am still attempting to do, with a few years of practice. Meanwhile if you, or they, want to develop the rotation scheme further, you should check out the book *Grow Your Own Vegetables* by the veg guru Joy Larkcom. In it, you'll find some fascinating tables with suggested planting regimes over several years. It might make an interesting alternative to a maths lesson.

Vegetable groups at a glance

1) **Potato** family includes: tomatoes, peppers, aubergines and … potatoes.
2) **Roots** include: parsley, parsnip, celeriac and fennel.
   Alliums include: onions, shallots, leeks and garlic.
   Beets include: beetroot, chard, perpetual spinach and spinach.
3) **Legumes** include: broad, French and runner beans, and peas.
4) **Brassica** family includes: cabbage, broccoli, kale, most of the oriental greens you are likely to encounter, salad rocket and – perhaps surprisingly – turnips and swede.

A three-year journal

Another innovation besides the raised beds was starting a journal. It would help us remember our planting for each rotation. You can make your own (see below) or buy one. I had been given a five-year gardener's 'record book' as a present, and thought this would be a good thing for the children to write up each week. It would be useful on busy days because I could set two of the older children the task of filling it in, theoretically freeing up more time to help the other children.

I say theoretically because it did not always work out like this. Depending on whose turn it was to fill in our journal, my scheme would sometimes backfire and I would spend a large part of the session explaining what to put in each of the columns. Still, all the children enjoyed this job, and accuracy did not matter too much – our journal entry for the first week of summer term helpfully informs the reader that lettuce and sunflowers are 'blooming'. In mid April? I doubt it. It was a way of getting them to think about what we were doing rather than just going through the motions, and I could always add my own version of events after each session.

Our very first entry, March 6 2007, reports a packed itinerary. It was sunny, though the ground was still 'very muddy'. That day, we potted on trailing petunias and gazanias bought as baby plug plants. (Potting on is literally that: moving the young plants into larger pots, where they would put on growth in the polytunnel before being moved outside in May.) We had also sown some tomato seeds and tobacco plants, though I don't recall the 'prooning' that is mentioned. It was still early spring, so the only flowering plants recorded around the school are 'daisys, daffidiles and dandielians'. It would get better.

How to make a three-year journal
It is very useful to be able to compare the same week in the garden, one year after another.

Specially designed record books are available for this, such as those published through the Royal Horticultural Society, but it feels more personal if children design their own and can customise it to suit your garden.

At its simplest, your record book/diary could be a strong, spiral-bound pad of A4 (I wouldn't use a smaller sized paper because you are aiming to create a table on each page). Turn the pad on to its side, so that you have a landscape view of it. Now, using a ruler, divide it into a table, first with three vertical lines, creating a narrow margin down the left-hand side of the sheet, and three more columns of roughly equal width.

Next, do your horizontal lines: you want three short columns at the top of the page, then three more columns on the remainder of the page.

Now fill in your table: working down from the top left corner, the left-hand margin should be divided into 'Date', 'Weather', 'What's happening in the garden' (this could be subdivided into as many different sections as you wish, such as 'Wildlife area', 'Veg patch', 'Pond' and so on), and 'What we did'. Now, fill in the date along the top. Let's say you are starting in Feb 2009: the first date should be 'Feb 2009, Week 1' then 'Feb 2010, Week 1' and finally 'Feb 2011, Week 1'.

During your first year, you will have to draw up a page as each week goes by, but the older children could take it in turns to do this, as well as filling in the book.

The alternative, of course, is to design a computer spreadsheet and get the children to fill that in each week in the classroom. But that loses the instantaneous appeal of a hard copy of a journal, with the different handwriting for each week, the grubby fingerprints and the battered cover. What could be more hands-on?

More on seed

With the polytunnel for germination and our one-and-a-half raised beds, our garden was taking shape. Every week in March we sowed more seed inside and some straight into the ground outside. Many of the children in gardening club this term were veterans of the previous summer, and remembered sowing seeds last time round. There was a feeling that many of us knew what we were doing; the vets could demonstrate an activity to the novices if I was distracted doing something else. We seemed to be developing a rhythm.

We would all squeeze into the polytunnel when it was raining or, when the weather improved, some would gather inside, some out, just like the plants. Conveniently, numbers would vary according to the conditions: when it was really bad, gardening club was cancelled anyway; in drizzle or damp, only a handful would turn up and we could usually all fit in the polytunnel; larger numbers usually reflected a pleasant day.

Outdoors, we sowed broad beans once again and early potatoes; indoors more broad beans (in order to compare rates of germination), Cos lettuce and tomatoes. As for flowers, we concentrated on sowing hardy annuals including sweet peas, cladanthus and, a little early perhaps, the half-hardy French marigolds and a lovely bronze-coloured annual rudbeckia, a relative of the popular yellow variety with its daisy-flower and blackish centre.

Some of the seeds were quick off the mark – notably the indoor broad beans and the lettuce – but others showed little sign of life. Our two seed trays of tomatoes in particular looked as though they would do nothing. They had been drenched so many times that a green moss was starting to form on the surface of the trays and I suspected they were done for. By the Easter holiday I had given up on them and left them on a shelf, only to find dozens of little seedlings greeting us on our return. Tomato plants expect lots of attention to grow correctly (*see page 146*), but their tiny seeds are clearly rather tough.

Still, it pays to treat your seed with respect. The first rule of seed sowing is to do what it says on the pack. However, some seed packets contain instructions that can be a little vague, some (aimed at an international audience) dispense with the written word and rely on graphics, while others assume a certain amount – too much in the case of children – of expertise.

Climate varies dramatically around the country, to say nothing of the way weather varies at any given time from year to year. In other words, one set of instructions is not a catch-all and rules are there for the bending. In such instances, then, it helps to have as great an understanding of your subject as possible. Here are a few thoughts that might make your seed sowing more successful.

- Most seed needs a soil temperature of 6°C to germinate.
- Though many seeds can be sown in situ, it often pays to give them a head start in a seed tray, placing it on a surface, indoors or out, depending on the time of year and instructions for germination. This is especially true if you

have a cold, wet, clay soil such as ours: seeds will benefit being started off inside, giving the earth outdoors a bit more time to warm up. Another reason to start seeds off in a tray is to keep seedlings well out of danger: it doesn't take long for a single marauding slug to massacre a sowing of young plants.

- After germination, be ruthless, thinning out seeds so they will not become overcrowded. The first time I did this in gardening club caused consternation among several children, to the extent that I began to doubt the wisdom of what I was doing. But be strong ... don't be tempted to leave them be as it will weaken the plants and could encourage infection (see damping off, below).

- It is best to sow seeds using both hands. First get the children to open the palm of one hand then sprinkle some seeds into it. Then, depending on the size of the seed and how close together they are sowing them, gather a few seeds or one at a time between the fingers of the other hand before sprinkling them on to the soil. This sounds so obvious, but I have never seen it written on any seed packet, and it is remarkable the number of times I have witnessed people pouring seeds straight from a packet on to the ground – adults as well as children.

- In an ideal world, most seedlings would prefer not to be disturbed and grow into strong, healthy plants in the exact place they were sown, but they can put up with the upheaval of transplanting. There are some, though, that absolutely hate to be moved. These are best sown where they are to flower or in long, thin 'root trainers' designed to minimise disturbance when seedlings are potted on or planted out. Alternatively, you can sow them in a good-sized pot or even the cardboard inside of a loo roll, which will break down in the soil over time. The pea family is a case in point, as are root crops such as carrot and parsnips. Poppies stand a good chance of failing if sown as seed to be transplanted.

- Salad leaf can be sown much more close together than recommended on the pack, then either thinned out as it begins to germinate, the thinnings making garnish for salads, or left to grow larger and used as a 'cut and come again' crop, typically harvested as immature, baby leaves when around 6cm high (see page 171). Plants that are good for this include lettuce, rocket, and Japanese greens such as red mustard and mizuna.

- Big seeds, such as sunflower, beans, nasturtiums and peas are easier for children to handle, so might govern your choice of plants to grow. In the chaos of a group sowing session, you are also more likely to see where they have ended up.

- If you are sowing straight outdoors, always sow in rows or some kind of regular pattern (zig zags or circles, say – ask the children what pattern they would like), so you can recognise the seedlings when they appear and distinguish them from weeds. Remember to put a stick at the end of each row to remind you exactly where your seedlings should appear. Let the children take it in turns to mark the rows with plastic plant labels.

- When sowing, after making an indentation, or drill, in the soil to take your seeds, water this first to encourage rooting.
- Few people have borders that are filled with a fine 'tilth', the term used to describe an ideal, crumbly soil with no clods of earth or stones in it. Tilth seems to exist only on gardening TV. So, when sowing outdoors, either cover seeds with general-purpose compost from the garden centre or get the children to sieve soil on to them using a riddle.
- Seeds sown in seed trays or modules with a polythene or glass covering often germinate more quickly than those without any covering. The covering helps to keep the compost moist. However, damp, warm conditions also encourage damping off, a common fungal disease. You can try to prevent this by good ventilation and by removing the covering as soon as germination occurs.
- Many gardeners advocate starting off their seeds in the airing cupboard, which acts like a heated propagator. Place damp newspaper on top of the trays to stop them drying out, and remove from the dark the moment they germinate.
- Always use tap water for seedlings, because the water butt might contain harmful fungal spores. Butt water is fine to irrigate established plants.
- Seed is relatively cheap but doesn't last forever so, if in doubt, chuck it out. During the spring term, some of the

children brought in seeds that their parents had given them (I suspect found in the bottom of a drawer) or, in some cases, from the outside of a cereal packet. Most of the seed I collected this way went unused. I had good reasons for this. First, a lot of the seed was out of date or of unknown provenance: had those packets that come with the cereal been stored correctly before they were paired off with the cornflakes? Second, it is important that you buy seed from a good supplier and that your seed is not too old, especially at a gardening club – when you have so little time, why risk planting things that might not germinate when reliable seed is inexpensive?

- Store seed in a cool, dark, dry place with the top of the packet sealed; an old biscuit tin is ideal.

- Having sown your seeds, water them with a fine rose. You don't want them being washed around the seedbed or tray every time they have a drink.

- Finally, don't be afraid to cheat. If you are only planning to grow a small amount, consider cutting out the potential heartache of failed germination and lost seedlings and buy in some baby plug plants instead.

In our second week of gardening club, and with some of the seeds that I had brought with me safely in their potting compost, I had asked the children to choose vegetables they would like to grow. The exercise soon turned into a competition to name something that no one else had thought of, and I began to doubt the effectiveness of this stab at democracy. But some names kept cropping up, such as courgettes, potatoes and carrots, so on to the list they went. I had my reservations about the latter, which are difficult to grow in our clay, but we would have a go. I had my own agenda, too, and gently hinted in the conversation at the veg that I thought would really suit us.

For me, the choice was relatively simple. I wanted species that were easy to cultivate, would fit in with a term-based timetable, would please the children in terms of quick-ish results, and that children were likely to eat, or at least taste. Some easy things, then, such as radish, I did not suggest: it is a complete doddle to grow, but I think it is horrible to eat and have yet to see a child consume one, so what was the point? Given the lack of space, I had my doubts about many of the slow-burn veg, too, such as cabbage, which would be sown in the spring and not harvested until late in the year.

Cabbage is not difficult to grow but, unlike another slow developer, the leek, is a real favourite of pests. Not only is it adored by caterpillars and pigeons, but it will need to get through the summer holidays with no one to water it. Also, if it does manage to survive until winter, it is really cheap in the shops. Surely a space is better used by concentrating on higher-value vegetables, especially if they are not too difficult to cultivate?

These ideas were not set in stone: they just helped us narrow down the list of what to grow. Any rules you set yourself can always be broken. For example, broad beans are one of *my* favourite vegetables to eat. Was it that wrong of me to impose my will? Just a little bit? No one had objected when we last sowed broad beans, and when they came up soon afterwards, the children were more excited than disappointed. It was the experience of growing that they really enjoyed. If they happened to like eating the vegetables, too, then so much the better.

What about flowers? Consulting the children on this subject looked like it would be even trickier because there is such a huge number to choose from. However, sunflowers, sweet peas and marigold were the names that popped up most frequently, so it was straightforward to expand from this base into other easy annuals that would be fun to grow from seed – nasturtiums, Love-in-a mist (*Nigella*) and cosmos were some of those that came to mind. We would grow some herbs too, especially basil.

Containers: the low-down

If you only have a small outside space, a container garden could be a good option for you. Containers are useful in any garden, because they can be moved around, hidden away when they are looking rough, or drafted in to pep up any part of the garden, be it the patio or flowerbed.

Most plants can be grown in a container, but their growth will be limited by the volume of the pot they are in. All the vegetables mentioned in this book are fine in a pot, though consideration should be given to size – potatoes and other roots need a decent depth to grow well and tall Jerusalem artichokes will be top-heavy and topple over if the pot is too small. Salad is a good crop to grow in a shallow container. Even trees can do well in a container, and there are plenty of 'dwarf' ornamental and fruit trees designed for the purpose.

All containers need to drain well, so should have a coarse material in their base – old stones, broken bits of pot or plastic are ideal; broken-up polystyrene packaging makes a good lightweight alternative. In a container of around 30cm diameter, aim to have your drainage material at a depth of at least 4cm. And it is often advisable to stand your pots on bricks, or 'feet' specially made for the purpose, so that the bottoms do not become waterlogged.

Typically, a container on sale at the garden centre will be made of terracotta or plastic, though it is possible to buy metal and wooden varieties and, of course, make your own from recycled objects. Terracotta is the good-taste option, but dries out more quickly than plastic and is heavier to move. You can alleviate the former problem by lining it with an old compost bag, remembering to puncture it with plenty of drainage holes first. Metal containers heat up and cool down quickly, meaning they will dry out more readily in the sunshine and anything planted in them could be more susceptible to the cold. Wooden containers will need to be made of oak, cedar or sweet chestnut, or treated so that they do not rot (try www.greenbuildingstore.co.uk for an eco-friendly preservative).

Soil in any pot will dry out more quickly than the soil in the garden, so will need to be watered regularly in summer, unless the weather is really wet (remember, however, that when pots are sited near buildings there will be a 'rain shadow' effect, and a shower could still leave them bone dry). You can help conserve water in a pot by a mulch of gravel to slow evaporation from the soil surface. Alternatively, you can plant drought-tolerant species. Ideal plants to survive dry conditions in a pot include Mediterranean herbs such as rosemary and thyme, and succulents such as sedum and sempervivum.

An easy meadow

The school had a largely hands-off approach to gardening club: there never seemed to be a problem with anything I wanted to do, as long as it did not intrude on curriculum time. The head teacher didn't have a problem with the construction of raised beds or our expanded gardening area, nor did they mind the coming and going of containers and hanging baskets in front of the school.

We planned to see if we could make a meadow. It sounds like a grand notion, but in reality a meadow can be created from a few square metres of ground. It makes an attractive feature in a garden, encourages insect wildlife such as butterflies, and at our gardening club was a great idea for the patch of grass by our polytunnel. It can be low maintenance, depending on the ground that you use (see below). You could be kept busy weeding out unwanted plants that try to colonise it, or you might be able to put your feet up as wildflowers, previously suppressed by regular mowing, finally get their day in the sun. You won't know until you have tried.

The type of meadow flowers and grasses you get will vary according to your soil conditions, but some general rules apply. The key to a successful meadow is to have rubbish soil, the sort of earth that has not been tended with fertilisers over the years. You want to mimic the poor soil that will encourage native grasses and flowers. Forget the characterless monocultural lawn that resembles a sitting-room carpet; you're aiming for the mix of the mongrel tomcat rather than thoroughbred Siamese. Such doctrine has led to meadow enthusiasts actually stripping off the topsoil to create the ideal conditions for wild plants and grasses to grow. This is for the zealots, however – such gardeners cut the flowers off their hostas to boost their foliage. I don't think you need to go to such extremes to get results. A corner of a playing field could be the perfect basis for a meadow.

Assuming you have identified your patch of ground and got the idea past the head teacher, what should you do next? Absolutely nothing. The grass should be left to grow after its final cut for winter, right through spring and summer to the following autumn. (There are other, more involved regimes, but this one I have found to work.) During this time, you should – *should* – get some interesting grasses and wildflowers springing up.

We put over to meadow a lozenge-shaped area around some young silver birches. The area is about 10 metres long and about four wide at its fattest point. Around its margin, the grass is kept mown, sending out a clear signal that the lozenge is deliberate and not some arbitrary patch of wilderness. If you wanted, you could also try mowing pathways through your meadow, to make the point that what you're looking at is design, not disarray. When the meadow gets its yearly cut, always rake off the mowings, giving them a week or so to dispatch their seed first, to stop them rotting and adding nutrients to the ground underneath. And never fertilise or feed – you want to starve your ground, not pamper it.

Our meadow is by no means spectacular, although there are several pretty grasses and flowering clovers. As time goes on, there is no reason why we won't add more plants to the mix, unless we want it to strictly mimic what might be found in the wild. Next autumn, for example, we might plant *Crocus tomassianus*, the best of the crocuses for naturalising in grass, for an early spring display. Daffodils could go in there too, their dying foliage being hidden by the grasses putting on a spurt of spring growth. Cammassia is a bulbous plant from the north American prairies that is planted in meadows. And I want to get hold of and try the delicate meadow scabious, which thrives nearby.

Just as you want to encourage interesting meadow plants, you should edit out those that look as if they are taking over. We pull up ragwort and try to catch the dandelions before they go to seed. If the meadow starts to become overwhelmed by other unwanted plants, such as dock and nettles, weed them out in the same way as you would a herbaceous border. If grass is taking over, crowding out wildflowers, yellow rattle is recommended by many meadow lovers because it is parasitic, weakening grasses and allowing more delicate species to come through. You can find this, together with other meadow seeds and advice, at Emorsgate (www.wildseed.co.uk) and Landlife (www.wildflower.org.uk).

Our meadow had its annual cut in late September and for two gardening club sessions after this, half the group raked and cleared the area, while the rest of us weeded the raised beds. It was perfect harvest weather, the grass yellowed and brittle under a mellow sun that had lost its summer blaze. Raking the meadow was the most popular activity, with the children taking it in turns to gather up the cuttings using some large plastic scoops that attach to your hands, like those novelty versions you see at football matches.

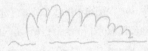

A garden for free

You don't need much to start a garden, just some containers, something to plant in them and soil or potting compost. Perhaps you might want seed trays, too, and a few small plant pots to get your seedlings going.

1) **Containers:** A container can be made from anything that will hold compost, be it a wellie or that classic recycled container, a tower of old car tyres (three is enough). It is best not to grow food in tyres, however, because of the chances of harmful residues leaching into the soil. At school, ask the kitchen for some of their old

catering-size tins; often these have bright logos that will look great lined up along a wall. And get students to bring in scrap to plant up – an old mop bucket, say, or broken wicker basket. Recycling is now encouraged in many municipal tips, so this could be a fertile hunting ground for suitable items such as old sinks and drainage pipes. It is important that the container has drainage, so remember to drill holes in its base if necessary. And if there is a chance of the soil being washed away (through the gaps in the old wicker basket, for example), line it first with an old compost bag, punching holes in it for drainage.

If you want to start seeds off indoors, you can use recycled materials instead of buying seedtrays and other potting paraphernalia. Get the children to bring in old yoghurt pots and the plastic trays used for fruit and veg at the supermarket: these are perfect for sowing seeds into, so long as they drain decently. Pricking out can be done with an old spoon.

Lastly, the cardboard inners of toilet rolls are a suitable replacement for root trainers designed for sowing seeds of plants that do not like their roots disturbed: when the seeds in them germinate, the whole thing can be planted out.

2) **Seeds:** With a bit of research finding free plants and seeds is possible. The Royal Horticultural Society's

Campaign for School Gardening (www.rhs.org.uk) provides free seeds for schools every year, while the Woodland Trust (www.woodland-trust.org.uk) does the same with hedgerow plants or young trees. The British Potato Council, meanwhile, promises to give seed potatoes to schools who register with them (www.potatoesforschools.org.uk).

3) The most difficult part of your free garden is finding decent **compost** to fill your containers. A 60-litre bag, enough to provide for half a dozen bucket-sized containers, could easily cost you £5. However, when our gardening club contacted our local garden centre, they were only too happy to get us going with compost, as well as young vegetable plants and flowers. Anecdotal evidence suggests this is not unique, so you should give it a go in your area: tempt them with a mention in the school's newsletter. If that fails, think big: there are loads of potential funding opportunities out there. A local bank might want to sponsor your gardening club, while B&Q runs 'Better Neighbour' grants to support community projects (www.diy.com).

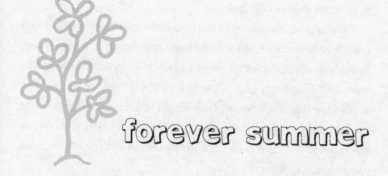

forever summer

It may be called summer term, but when school returns after the Easter break, it is best to not get your hopes up with dreams of eternal sunshine. At this time of year – usually mid-April – anything can happen with the weather, from warm showers to cold snaps and hail.

Our summer term, however, was ushered in by a fabulously hot Easter that surely spooked those who were taking climate change seriously. Personally, I was filled with optimism for the weeks to come, as well as relief that I had organised a watering rota during the holiday.

Watering

At the end of the previous term, I had singled out a few children who I knew lived near the school and whose parents I thought would not mind a turn at watering over the holiday. The children had a vested interest in hassling their parents (dead plants, otherwise). The adults could be relied on to write down or remember the specific dates.

I calculated that to cover the two-week break, we needed four families. My children had already been press-ganged into helping, so we now needed another three. Each family would do at least two days with a one-day gap in between shifts. If they could commit to another day, even better. That would be enough if the weather stayed nice and the polytunnel doors remained open so as not to get too hot. If it took a turn for the worse, then their instructions were to stay at home.

Stock control

While the watering rota had kept the plants healthy during the holidays, their immediate future was less secure. In the polytunnel, most of the surfaces, including part of the floor, were now covered in pots and trays of seedlings queuing up to go in the ground. The nasturtiums and French marigolds were doing well, but we would keep them indoors for a little longer – just to make sure that they didn't get caught by a late frost. The sunflowers were just about ready for the children to take home, so that would be one group of polytunnel dwellers that now had somewhere to go.

Meanwhile, a large box full of plug plants was delivered to us in early May, after we had signed up to a scheme offering free veg seedlings to primary schools. Soon after that, Mrs B, one of the lunchtime staff, gave us a couple of dozen red cabbage plants and purple sprouts for a matching border of brassicas. By the time the remaining topsoil arrived, in the second week of the month, we had more than enough young plants to fill up our new garden.

If spring term is one of new beginnings, of sowing crops and making plans for our brief gardening season, summer is about consolidation. We started off more crops this term, but a large part of it would be bringing on what we had already got into the garden. That, and perhaps the best bit – the harvest.

Early summer term, then, is a time to do something with all the seedlings you have raised, whether it's thinning, potting on, hardening off or planting out – or a combination of all of them. It means that our sessions became more varied with much more to cram in. But what do all these expressions mean?

Thinning

When seeds germinate they need space to grow, and don't want competition for water and nutrients from other seedlings. Thinning, then, simply means removing weaker seedlings in an overcrowded seed tray, giving the strongest more room. A useful tip is not to uproot the seedlings you are thinning out, because this might disturb the roots of those you wish to keep. Instead, snip them with a pair of scissors and remove.

Pricking out

Moving seedlings into a larger container or bed, say from seed trays into individual pots to allow them more space to grow, is known as pricking out. Seedlings are generally ready to be moved

83

when two proper leaves have formed. When moving seedlings, hold them gently by the leaf, not the stem, and try to take as much root with you as possible, preferably with the compost intact around it; you can get tiny little shovels to help you do this, or you can use the end of a plant label. Make a hole in the compost where the seedling is to go, drop it in, gently firm the compost around the base of the plant, and water. Keep out of direct sunshine for a couple of days. Pricking out is unnecessary when seeds have been sown into individual modules.

Potting on

Moving potted plants to larger pots, or modules, to continue growing is known as potting on. You would do this with any plants you intend to grow indoors, such as tomatoes; or when a plant outgrows its pot but is either not ready to go outside because the conditions are not right (plant too small; soil or weather too cold). You want your plant to have a good root system and you can usually tell this by easing the plant from its pot; if the compost holds together, there is a healthy root system and it is ready to move on. Now, gently tip the plant out of its pot and, cupping the rootball and surrounding compost in your hands, move it to its new home.

Planting out

The same rules apply as for potting on. If the compost of the plant is dry, water first. If it is bone dry, it might be best to soak the pot for an hour or two before the plant goes in the ground. Sometimes, with perennials bought from the garden centre, the compost can be so dry that it is worth soaking the plant overnight, to make sure the potting medium rehydrates. Once you have made the hole in which the plant is to go, fill it with water before planting. This will help roots to grow downwards rather than look for moisture towards the soil surface.

Hardening off

Plants that have been raised indoors need to be acclimatised to the real weather out in the garden over a period of two to three weeks. Once they are used to the lower temperatures and increased air movement, they can be planted out. Hardening off is a gradual process, usually practised with tender or half-hardy plants such as French marigolds. It can be quite an involved process, using cold frames, a greenhouse and the outdoors, but I am assuming you only have two options – indoors and out.

There is no precise formula, but use your common sense. French marigolds, for example, will be planted out when all risk of frost has passed (the second week of May is a good rule of thumb, but it will depend where you live). Start off by leaving the plants outside in a sheltered spot for a short period each day. Then leave them out all day, bringing them in at night. Eventually the seedlings can be left out all the time (unless a very cold night is forecast), and at this point they are ready to plant out.

Of course, this is the ideal scenario, one that is difficult to put into practice if you are not in school all day. For us, hardening off involved me leaving the plants outdoors in the mornings when I brought my children to school (or asking my wife to do this if she was dropping off the children), then asking whoever was on watering rota to bring them in at lunchtime. After a while they would be left out all day, for me to bring in when I picked my daughters up at 3.30pm.

If bad weather was forecast, the plants would simply stay in the polytunnel, with one of the doors open all the time. It is another of those gardening tasks for which you develop a feel. Cold snap? Leave them in the polytunnel. Freezing? Close the door, too. Very hot? Leave them out all day.

The hosepipe bans

As the one-and-a-half raised beds turned into two, and two into three, and the sun continued to shine, keeping all the plants watered became more of an issue. It was around this time I eventually relented and let the children use the hosepipe. Up until now, with only seedlings to water in the polytunnel and little over a quarter of our outside garden functioning, they had taken it in turns to fill watering cans at the outside tap (about half full, far too heavy otherwise) and carry them the 15 metres or so back.

Now, though, with our plants and patch expanding, together with the heat, it made sense to have water closer to our base. We would trail the hosepipe over to the raised beds, turn the tap to a steady flow, and fill up watering cans from there. In between cans, the hose would rest in a raised bed so no water was wasted, and get moved from time to time so that other bits of the ground got a drink.

On gardening club days, our watering took place at the most inefficient time possible, when the sun was at its highest, and some of the water would evaporate. But this was the only way to ensure everyone in gardening club got to do this most favoured of activities. The daily watering rota that we had started the previous summer was only open to the older students.

A real live hosepipe proved a temptation too far for some of the children, and in between filling watering cans it was constantly picked up, put down, sprinkled on the ground. We were not setting a good example for sensible use of this most precious resource but in the interests of fair play, I did not think it too bad, especially as it was only once a week. It only became a problem if someone made a jet from the hose by putting their thumb over the end, which could then dislodge young plants if sprayed directly at them.

Annie was the worst culprit and though I am sure she never intended to do so, she nearly always ended up watering anyone near her as well as the plants. She just couldn't get the hang of turning her head round without moving her body, too, including the hand that was holding the hose. It would go something like this. 'Don't spray the garden, Annie, you might kill the plants,' someone would say, at which point, Annie would swivel round to see who had spoken to her, the hose still in her hand and an arc of water spraying anyone who was in the way. Complain and she would turn back to see who was shouting at her, again wetting anyone in her path. The scene was pure panto.

Slugs, snails and other foes

Early summer term brings with it a genuine sense of renewal in the garden. Herbaceous beds are alive with bulbs and thickening with summer perennials ... buds and blossom cover the shrubs and trees. All around you get the impression that nature is on the move – and that, alas, means slugs and snails, too, the unspeakable in pursuit of the edible.

Gardeners – and I suspect many non-gardeners, too – are driven to near madness by them. They provoke extremes of behaviour in otherwise balanced people, such as going out at night, armed with a torch and a sharp or blunt weapon, like some green-fingered vigilante.

The destructive abilities of slugs and snails are legendary. Just look at the callousness with which they operate. Why, for example, are they not content to nibble through a few leaves, eat their fill and continue on their way? Instead, like some terrible army with a scorched-earth policy, they sever the stem of a plant and leave the rest of it to die.

One way that the green-minded gardener can combat slugs and snails is to encourage their natural predators such as hedgehogs, birds and frogs into the garden. At school, our garden is surrounded by a nice chunky hedgerow – home to birds and maybe a hedgehog – and early in the summer term I was lulled into thinking that this would be enough to keep the pests in check. Early plantings out from the polytunnel suffered few casualties, and an outdoor sowing of rocket grew untouched. Clearly something living in the hedge was on our side ...

At first, my do-nothing strategy worked – whether because of the proximity of the hedgerow or the exceptionally dry conditions through April I'll never know. By early autumn, however, the pests were rampant. The red cabbage and purple sprouts lay in tatters. I should have known better. Take your eye off the ball for a minute and the slugs and snails will make you pay. With interest.

It is tempting, when surveying the damage wrought by these creatures, to go nuclear and reach for the worst kind of chemical deterrent you can find. However, there are three main ways to combat slugs and snails:

1) First, know your enemy and take evasive action – prevention is better than cure.
2) Get others to do the work for you – encourage natural predators.
3) When all else fails – you've tried deterrence, sanctions, too – go on the attack yourself.

Know your enemy

Snails and slugs need places to hide – under rocks, in piles of rotting vegetation or in long grass. They adore cool, wet conditions and shade, hate hot, dry conditions and glaring sunshine. Any rotting veg will also be a food source – this is fine on the compost heap but old leaves decaying next to a lettuce will initially attract them to the area. It is then only a matter of time before they realise what a good thing they are on to and start on your healthy veg. The moral here is to be tidy in your garden, at least around your plants.

Yes, have wild bits that will encourage predators to feed on these pests, but maybe not right next door to your prize plants.

Snails seem to be more of a pest in the city, perhaps because they have nice cool garden walls in which to hide. When we lived in London, a night-time visit to the garden was like a horror movie, dozens – maybe hundreds, I couldn't bear to count – of snails heading from the old brick wall on one side of the garden, across the patio towards the flowerbeds.

Many slugs live underground, so don't think you are ever safe. Like snails, they are creatures of the night: if you want to get the true measure of their numbers, go outside when it's dark.

Defeat your enemy

Slugs and snails hate copper – it reacts with their slime, purportedly giving them a mini electric shock when they touch it – and you can buy various copper-based 'barriers' from the garden centre, including rings to go round the base of plants and mats that sit under plant pots. However, this can get expensive if you have a lot of pots to protect. Make sure also that none have been trapped inside the barrier – otherwise, it kind of defeats the object.

A much cheaper but arguably less aesthetic alternative is to cut the bottoms and tops off clear plastic drinks bottles and put the resulting cylinder around young plants. It will act as a mini cloche, too, protecting the plant from the worst of the weather.

There are many other proprietary and home-made barriers, which include sharp, spiky materials that are difficult to slither over, such as gravel and grit. Get the children to bring in suitable materials from home and try out their effectiveness. These might include old crushed eggshells, wood ash, coffee grounds, pine needles and bran. The latter also reacts with slugs when they eat it, causing them to bloat up and die. For plants in pots, smear a ring of Vaseline around the rim, which slugs or snails will not cross. Meanwhile, some gardeners swear by crushed garlic, added to water and sprinkled around vulnerable plants. Like those other creatures of the night, vampires, slugs can't stand it.

The problem with many barriers, however, is they get gradually washed away by rain and will need topping up in wet weather – the time when slugs and snails are at their most dangerous. And with any barriers, make sure there are no overhanging objects or foliage that the creatures can use as a bridge to their intended prey.

Another way to prevent slugs and snails getting the better of you is to raise healthy plants. A strong, vigorous young plant has more chance of surviving mollusc attacks than a weakling that struggles on the best of days. This is one good reason for sowing seedlings indoors or in trays that are raised up off the ground – your plants get a head start and are bigger when they go out to face the dangers of the wider world.

Unless you are growing for a specific purpose, such as vegetables to eat, why bother having plants that are prone to slug and snail attacks in the first place? Generally speaking, slugs and snails are not interested in plants with hairy foliage, leathery leaves and a strong scent.

Some popular plants that slugs seem to avoid:

Flowers: Perennial geraniums, foxgloves, sea holly and other thistly kin, daffodils, nasturtiums, snowdrops and calendula.

Vegetables: Onions, garlic, lamb's lettuce, tomatoes, beetroot, red lettuce, most herbs (clearly they don't like the strong taste) and peppery salads such as rocket and Japanese mustard. Some varieties of potato are more slug resistant than others, so check when buying seed potato.

Natural predators

A wildlife garden is the perfect way to encourage natural predators. Birds, frogs, toads, slowworms and hedgehogs number among the creatures who eat snails, slugs or both. Apparently, a hedgehog can get through 120 slugs an hour.

Due to their difference in size, ground beetles and centipedes are perhaps less obvious slug and snail predators but don't underestimate them. Ground beetles will also attack caterpillars and aphids.

Offensive measures

When slugs and snails seem to be getting the better of you, despite the preventive measures and predators you have drafted in, it is time to go on the offensive.

A simple, though extremely effective tactic is to go out in the dark with a torch and gather up, or kill, all the slugs and snails you can find (I'll come to how to dispose of them in a minute). The best time to do this is a couple of hours after sunset, though in the warmer months, when these creatures are at their most active, this could get rather late. This presents two problems. First, can you really be bothered to schlepp down to the school at such a time? Second, how do you explain what you are doing should a policeman or security guard happen by, especially if you are carrying a blunt or sharp instrument to kill the snails and slugs.

Given this, perhaps other methods are more suitable for the school garden. Regular hoeing of your cultivated area, for example, is very effective, as it brings slugs and their eggs to the surface of the soil, exposing them to predators.

Nematode worms are another means of control. These are parasites that attack slugs and are, some gardeners claim, effective against snails, too. Usually only available by mail order, they will arrive packed in clay (try www.greengardener.co.uk or www.organic catalog.com). Mix the nematodes with water in a watering can and sprinkle the affected ground.

Nematodes are extremely effective, and the great thing about them is you do not have to dispose of any bodies – the slugs crawl back into the soil or their hiding places to die. Nematodes do, however, have their drawbacks. For a start, at around £10 to treat an area of 40m^2, they are expensive. Secondly, they require certain conditions to work properly. The soil has to be at least 5°C and moist but not soaking: very dry or very wet weather could hinder their ability to perform. Thirdly, one dose of nematodes will not leave you safe for the whole season: they last for up to six weeks, at which time you will have to apply them again.

Slug traps

A simpler and cheaper method of catching snails and slugs is to get the children to make their own traps. This can simply be an upturned pot or tile that is near some vulnerable plants. Slugs and snails will congregate underneath here to take advantage of its cool, dark environment. In the morning, gather up the molluscs before it gets too hot and they look for somewhere else to hide. You can do the same thing with an upturned, scooped-out half of grapefruit, melon or orange. Always remember to leave a gap between the soil and the trap so that the creatures can get inside. If you can, try to get some children to meet you in the garden just before school; then you can see what you have trapped and which method works best.

Slightly more complicated, but very effective, is the slug pub. You'll need a plastic pot with a lid, and some slug-and-snail sized slots cut into the rim, like the crenellated walls on a castle. A large yoghurt pot should do the trick. Sink the pot into the ground, leaving 3cm of it sticking out of the soil. This is to stop ground beetles falling in. Now, put some bait into the pot. Typically, people use beer, but milk, grape juice, even jam mixed with water will do. Now put the lid back on and return the next day to see what you have caught overnight. It is important that you put the lid on: the latter will prevent the rain getting in, diluting your bait or flooding the pot; it will also slow down evaporation and it will stop beneficial creatures such as frogs drinking it.

To catch a thief

Once you've trapped your slugs and snails, how do you dispose of them if they are still alive? Some gardeners have no qualms about crushing them or cutting them in half (hence the hammer and the scissors on those nightly patrols) but I am too squeamish for this. Occasionally, I have crushed snails under bricks, at the same time taking care to look away, but don't feel this is something to share with children.

At school, when we do find slugs or snails, we chuck them on the compost heap or into the hedgerow nearby and hope something will come along to deal with them. I have no idea whether the former solution works, although it is popular with some organic gardeners: slugs and snails are actually more partial

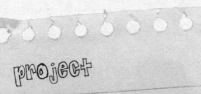

project

The best bait

Make several slug traps out of yoghurt pots and try different baits in each of them (see above). Now leave them overnight. The next day, count how many slugs and snails you have caught. Is one bait more effective than another? Do slugs prefer beer to milk? Can you think why?

to rotting vegetation than the fresh stuff, but the worry is that it could get a bit crowded in the compost heap, leaving some of them to explore potential food sources elsewhere. The latter means of disposal, meanwhile, could possibly be foolish. Slugs and snails are reputed to have a homing instinct, leaving a scented trail behind them so that they can find their way back in the dark. Disposing of them too close to your garden could merely be prolonging the problem.

Some gardeners advocate suffocating snails and slugs in a carrier bag; some that they should be drowned in a bucket of salty water. Others, meanwhile, suggest they be given more humane treatment and taken to a field or wasteland, well away from any gardens, and released.

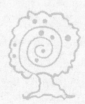

Other common pests

Aphids

There are hundreds of different types of aphid, but blackfly and greenfly are the most common. The easiest – and greenest – way to get rid of them is to brush them off a plant, or spray them with a fine jet of water. The less squeamish children find this a satisfying task. Soft soap is a pesticide made from natural products and allowed under organic principles. Derris dust is permitted too, but kills beneficial insects as well as the baddies. But do you really need a pesticide for aphids? Organic growers prefer such things as a last resort only. A more natural solution could be planting: chives, planted around a vulnerable crop will deter aphids, while the likes of the poached egg plant *Limnanthes douglasii* will attract ladybirds and hoverflies, by far the best natural control.

Red spider mite

These are a problem with plants raised indoors, covering them with a fine web and leaving foliage yellow and dessicated. Keep the air humid to deter them.

Flea beetle

These make tiny holes in young plants and are most prevalent in the warmer months of the summer. They are a particular nuisance with rocket and Oriental greens, which is a good reason for growing these plants either side of the summer, when they are less active. Growing a crop under horticultural fleece keeps them at bay, too. Other vulnerable plants include turnips and swede.

New pests on the block

The harlequin ladybird, which arrived in Britain in 2004, has a voracious appetite for aphids; the problem is that it does not stop there. Harlequins, according to the Royal Horticultural Society (RHS), also eat beneficial insects such as hoverfly larvae, lacewings and (worst) native ladybirds. They can have several different markings: all are slightly bigger than the native ladybird, which you'll recognise because it has seven spots. If it has more spots or is black with red spots, beware: you're probably looking at a harlequin.

Other new arrivals to Britain that have made the RHS top ten pests (slugs and snails are number one, of course) are the rosemary beetle, berberis sawfly and the horse chestnut leaf-mining moth, which causes severe browning of the leaves of conker trees.

Pest control for free

To keep the pests under control, use the help of some good guys. Here's the top ten – with their menu preference:

1. **Ladybird:** Attract with plant pollen and nectar-rich plants. Likes to overwinter in nooks and crannies, such as around the window frame of a shed and inside bamboo canes. Eats aphids.
2. **Hoverfly:** Likes similar conditions to ladybirds. Eats spider mites, while the hoverfly larva eats aphids and mites.
3. **Lacewing:** Enjoys similar conditions to hoverflies and ladybirds. (See page 212 for how to make a winter hotel for lacewings, hoverflies and ladybirds.) Eats mites and caterpillar larvae.
4. **Ground beetle:** Lives in soil and piles of rotting leaves. Eats slugs and vine weevil.
5. **Frogs and toads:** Enjoy long grass, neglected corners. Frogs prefer damp conditions and ponds. Toads like a drier hideaway. Eat slugs and snails.

6. **Wasp:** It is not a good idea to have a lot of them in a school garden. Likes nectar rich plants. Eats caterpillars and spider mites.

7. **Hedgehog:** Enjoys hedgerows, old leaf piles and wood piles. Can eat up to 100 slugs, caterpillars and insect larvae in one night.

8. **Slowworm:** Like a warm place such as an undisturbed compost heap, or underneath a piece of corrugated metal roofing left in the sun. Extremely fond of slugs.

9. **Blue tit:** Partial to an ordinary garden feeder. Particularly fond of black sunflower seeds. Eats aphids – will snack on these while waiting it's turn on the feeder.

10. **Thrush:** Leave bits of apple on the lawn to tempt it into the garden. Alas, rare these days, but when it appears, there is no better expert at cracking and eating snails.

Salad at the school gates

It was a great day when we fed the whole school with potatoes. Our modest planting was enough for two separate sittings. The firm, white scrapers that came out of the earth nailed the ghost of the rotten crop the previous year. Several harvests of French beans would follow, proper veg from a proper garden, and what with picking, watering and weeding the second half of term flew by.

Not everything we grew that summer ended up in the school kitchen's pot. By the middle of term, we were heading for a glut of lettuce and the rocket needed harvesting before it went to seed in the heat. The school cook and I had formed an uneasy alliance about what she would and wouldn't take from the kitchen garden, so I knew not to push my luck. Salad might go down well in some places right through summer. But in a rural kitchen that fed primary-school children? Somehow I doubted it.

But what about selling salad after school? The children thought this a great idea, the only question now being exactly how to do it. Our first attempt was an honesty box under the shade of a tree near the school gate. A few of the older children got permission to join me during afternoon break in the garden, where we picked some lettuce, packed them neatly into one of those wide, shallow fruit boxes from the supermarket, then left it resting at an angle under the tree. Beside it, we left an honesty box – a small biscuit tin that has since become the gardening club treasury – with a note advertising the price: 30p, five pence more than that being sold by the elderly man at the end of the road. But ours were mighty Webb's Wonderful lettuce, his the soft-leaved butterhead that would only make one meal and wilt if not eaten the same day. We hoped that parents would appreciate the difference and as the school drifted out at 3.30pm, we stood to one side and waited.

The lettuce sold badly at the school gates, but did not go to waste. As the last of the children and their parents dispersed, any gardening club members remaining took a plant each home. I bought a couple myself – excellent value for organically grown salad – and distributed the rest among a grateful staffroom. It was disappointing nevertheless: we should advertise ourselves better, maybe get out there among the punters, hawking our wares.

A few weeks later, we had more lettuce and some rocket to sell, and this time set up a table outside the main entrance. Annie and Eldest daughter volunteered to look after our little shop, with its neat pile of freezer bags, its large healthy box of fresh leaf and its biscuit-tin till. Despite their best efforts at scaring people off by shouting out prices and 'Come and get it!', the rocket sold out before the rest of the children were let out of class. The lettuce soon followed and we were cleaned out in a matter of minutes.

Next time, though, we should advertise ourselves more and bolt ourselves on to one of the fundraisers that the school runs on Friday afternoons from time to time. Next time, we also intend to have more to sell than rocket and lettuce.

Making a pond

Ponds are a tricky subject in the context of a school, because of the obvious safety issues surrounding them. I know of one school that filled in its pond because it was felt that a pond was too dangerous for the children.

This is a pity, because a pond is a magnet for wildlife as well as children. A pond attracts many beneficial creatures – frogs, for example – who don't need any invitation to colonise it and will move in almost overnight. But not only are ponds good for the garden and wildlife, they offer tremendous potential for educational activities such as pond dipping.

There are several ways to make a pond or water feature safe enough for children, so don't rule one out immediately.

If you want a fully-fledged pond, one solution is to fence it off from the rest of the school, with access via a latched gate; this could either be padlocked or with the latch high enough so that young children cannot reach it. Another soluion is to fit a galvanised steel grille over the pond at the same level as the water surface. This can be concealed by large pebbles placed on top and with plants growing through it and at the margins.

Another alternative is to make a pond from an old barrel or a sink. Plants can be suspended by wire secured at the edge to the appropriate depth, or rested on a submerged platform. If doing this, make sure that there is a slope at one side of the pond, so that creatures can get in and out of it. A pile of stones or a piece of wood to act as a ramp will do.

Perhaps you do not need a pond after all: a boggy area with stepping stones through it will attract all manner of wildlife and can be planted up with marginals (see below) that will thrive in such conditions.

Ultimately, what kind of pond you have will depend on budget. It could get expensive, for example, fencing off an area, and a metal grille will need solid sides to rest on – this might also prove too formal for what you had in mind.

Positioning of your pond is vital. It is important that the pond is not too close to a hedged boundary or trees, otherwise it will get clogged up with autumn leaves. A nearby hedge, however, will provide important shelter, but try to position the pond in an open sunny site where it is not overhung by trees or shrubs.

How to build a pond

It is best to build a pond in autumn or spring, when it will be filled up with rainwater. Filling a pond with tap water only stores up trouble for you in the future, because any nutrients in the water are more likely to encourage algal growth. Never introduce fish: they will only gobble up the rest of the wildlife.

You will need

- pond liner (see below for quantity)
- spade
- purpose-built fibre matting, old carpet (not foam-backed), flooring underlay or old newspapers
- builder's sand: enough to cover the base of your pond to about 6cm depth

Mark out the site of your pond and the shape (using a hose, or a line of sand, or pegs pushed into the ground at intervals).

Now get digging. A pond should be at least 60cm deep in the middle so that creatures can retreat here from extremes of temperature, but it is important that at least one side is a shallow gradient, so amphibians can easily get in and out of the water. A shelf around the edge of the pond will mean you can plant 'emergent' species here.

Once you have dug your hole, remove any sharp stones and roots: this will help to ensure the pond liner does not get punctured in future. The length of liner needs to be the proposed length of the pond plus twice the depth; similarly the width needs to be the width of the pond plus twice the depth. Flexible liners (as opposed to rigid plastic or fibreglass) come in various materials and quality; the best is butyl rubber, the thicker the better.

Before you put in the liner, shovel sand about 6cm deep into the hole, then put the underlay material on top. This will help to prevent the liner getting punctured. Allow for about 10cm of liner overlap at the edge of the pond, so that it can be buried in the ground around the pond.

Now wait … the rain will fill it up.

What to plant

Although a pond can be built any time in the autumn or spring, it is best planted between April and September. Planting in a pond is crucial: many creatures that thrive in ponds do so because there is a habitat for them: open water simply exposes them to predators.

Unfortunately, it is not always the best idea to pop down to the garden centre and buy whatever is on sale there. There are many so-called pond plants that, given half the chance, turn into raving beasts that take over your pond to the exclusion of other species and life. Some of these have escaped into waterways and now plague streams and ditches. Australian swamp stonecrop or New Zealand pygmy weed (*Crassula helmsii*), for example, has spread widely in garden centres and nurseries and has often seeded in the pots of other bought plant stock. Other plants to avoid are water fern (*Azolla filiculoides*) and parrot's feather (*Myriophyllum aquaticum*).

Many garden centres are wise to this, but foreign plants that are not suited to our environment still slip through the net. It is important to check your sources well.

The Pond Trust (www.brookes.ac.uk/pondaction), which provides advice on establishing a wildlife pond, advocates simply leaving your pond alone: eventually plants that are most suited to your site will colonise, along with appropriate creatures. Failing that, it says, you should try to use local plants to maintain the natural distinctiveness, biodiversity and gene pool of wetland species in your local area.

Plants for ponds can be divided into three categories:

1) True **aquatics** are a small group that have their roots underwater; with some, such as water lilies, their leaves come to the surface. Generally, these plants grow only in still water. They include water lilies, oxygenating weeds (eg potamogeton and starwort) and sweet-scented water hawthorn, *Aponogeton distachyos*. Note: if you plant a waterlily, be warned that some are very vigorous. More manageable waterlilies are cultivars of *Nymphea odorata*. To plant an aquatic, put the pot into a mesh basket with gravel over the top of the compost to keep the compost in place, then lower into the pond. Stones placed around the base of the basket will help to keep the basket in place. Ideally, you should aim for about two thirds of the pond covered in plants, and one third open water.

2) Towards the water's edge are the **emergents**. These are planted where the water and ground meet – some grow out on to land, some into water. Examples include all the reed family, such as the tall Norfolk reeds and iris.

3) **Marginal** plants sit on the riverbank and like damp roots. Many herbaceous plants are happy in this situation. Familiar faces include loosestrife and thalictrum. Butterbur is another (so called because its large leaves were used to wrap butter).

Pond maintenance

Your pond should not need much maintenance, apart from the occasional clear-out of fallen leaves. It is best to do this in early autumn, away from the breeding season and before any animals have gone into hibernation. Always leave some debris at the bottom of the pond, however.

In summer, remove excess blanket weed by twisting it round a stick. Duckweed can be scooped out with a sieve. Always leave the weed on the pondside overnight, so that any creatures in there can get back to their home.

In dry periods, the pond might need a top-up with tap water. Always do this in small amounts, so changes in temperature or chlorine levels do not have an adverse effect.

You'll find more information at www.froglife.org.

project

How many different creatures can you see in your pond? A wildlife pond might contain the following: frogs, toads, diving beetles, water boatmen, water skaters, water measurers, damselflies, dragonflies, water snails and, if you are lucky, newts.

The village show

Our annual village show is every bit the traditional rural event, the sort of thing you read about and see in TV dramas but never quite believe to be true. There is a prize for the heaviest marrow, and a flower section where roses and dahlias dominate. A category is devoted to strawberry jam and there is one for the best plate of fudge. The vegetable section, meanwhile, has four out of 27 categories devoted to the onion family and two to the marrow. If it were not for the photography competition, you would think it was the 1950s.

Earlier in the year, the secretary of this committee contacted me to ask if there should be a school category in the show. It was a nice idea, I thought, but not the right timing. Seeing that the event falls in the middle of the summer holidays, I was not sure how it would work.

I suppose I was being lazy, too. At the back of my mind I imagined the end of the summer term in July when the responsibility of keeping all our produce healthy for the August event would fall on to me. Imagine if something died in my charge or I didn't get round to watering on a particularly hot day!

Anyway, I had never been entirely enthusiastic about this competition. I find the old-fashionedness too much. It enforces stereotypes and peddles the idea that big is always better than flavour. A prize for the heaviest marrow? Surely this harks back to the time, post-war, when you would eke as much as you could from your veg patch to supplement rations. The more massive your marrow, the more food there was to eat, regardless of the fact that it was tasteless and watery. To pick that marrow instead as a young, sweet courgette, the thinking went, was to squander its potential. But rationing ended 50 years ago. When I once proposed to a committee member that there might be an organically grown category I might as well have suggested strippers. It was a true tumbleweed moment.

But by early August and with the date of the show approaching, I was beginning to change my tune. It was my first full season with the gardening club, and I was quietly proud of what we had achieved. Nothing wrong with entering on their behalf, I told myself, and it would be wonderful for the children to win something for what they had grown.

I had my eye in particular on the amazing French beans the wet summer had produced. All through the holidays, some of the children who lived near the school had been picking these lovely veg and taking them home to their families, which only made the plants produce more.

There were boisterous clumps of French marigolds, too, whose yellow flowerheads flecked with chocolatey brown were now in their second flush but still looking beautiful. The sweet peas had become such a thicket of mauve- and cream-coloured blooms that the frame we built for them had collapsed. There was a chocolate annual rudbeckia that I had given up for dead but had revived itself in the rain, and courgettes and parsley. All this yet, save for the French-bean harvesters, no one to appreciate it. Maybe there was no harm entering a few things from the gardening club, after all. At least the wider village would get to see what we were up to.

All entries had to be received by 10.30am sharp, so I was at school early that Saturday morning. I thought about ringing round some of the gardening club, to see if they wanted to help, but seeing that I couldn't even get my own girls out of their pyjamas and away from the TV at that time, I decided not to bother. The deadline stipulated that everything had to be laid out according to the show's instructions, with the entry form filled in and entries placed in the correct part of the hall. There was no room for manoeuvre: mistakes would not be tolerated. The previous year, we had watched a flustered lady rush into the building with a gorgeous display of homemade cakes, only to be turned away because she was five minutes late. And a friend's child had her offering of sweet peas disqualified because there were too many blooms in the bunch. Exceptions cannot be made when the stakes are a prize at the village show.

The school had five entries in the show, and I returned after lunch with other local hopefuls to see how we had done. Nothing for our sweet peas. Was it because my bunch was not 'mixed' enough as the category stated, being only two subtle variations on the same colour? Or was it the fact that in my panic to get everything sorted by 10.30am, I had left them in a jar instead of the white vase I had brought with me. The 'five sprigs of parsley' and marigolds scored a similarly disappointing blank, and I consoled myself that it was because of their presentation and nothing to do with their quality. We got a 'highly commended' in the novice collection of three vegetables for a courgette, sprig of parsley and French bean. As for our collection of 'five beans, with no podding showing through the skin' ... first prize!

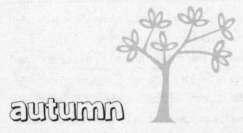

autumn

After a really disappointing summer, so wet it no doubt broke some kind of meteorological record, it seemed that the weather was anxious to please us after ruining the holidays. A long dry spell and mild, sunny days made it feel as though the colourful but usually brief turning of the hedges and trees would go on for ever.

The wet summer and mild autumn also meant that when the children returned to school, the garden still had lots to offer. The sweet peas, tagetes and the wonderful bronze rudbeckia were set to continue until the first frosts. I think I was more excited by this than the children. Every Tuesday I enthused that these beautiful plants (the rudbeckia in particular was stunning) had been grown by them, from seed, only a few months before. By way of reply, I would get slightly baffled looks, or an almost inaudible 'Yep'. As if they did this sort of thing every day.

Weeds, weeds, weeds

While the flowers had been thriving, however, so had the weeds in all the empty spaces left in the garden. Six weeks of neglect had turned our raised beds into a paradise for dock, sow thistles and nettles. The list of offenders also included a clump of self-seeded pink poppies. They were pretty enough, but their flowering is brief and their seed heads, if left alone, would only mean more trouble to come.

Looking over our four raised beds, it was obvious we had broken one of the golden rules of weed control – we had let them run to seed over the summer, when perhaps we could have been more vigilant towards the end of term. Now, in the soil in which we wanted to grow things next season were thousands of dormant seeds, guaranteeing that we would be kept busy in the spring – and that was even before we cleared this lot. There is a saying: one year's seeding, seven years' weeding. If this is true, these children would almost be applying for university by the time this patch was under control.

I was surprised to find that many of the children at gardening club loved weeding. I thought they would see it as the gardening equivalent of washing-up: tried once, then only repeated when bribed or under duress. Certainly my own children had never shown much enthusiasm for it. Perhaps its appeal, however, is that it's one of the jobs where you can to some extent leave them to it. There is not much harm to be done, as long as you first point out the plants that you're not trying to get rid of.

A weed is anything you don't want in the garden, be it a pest that strangles other plants such as ground elder, or a popular flower that has seeded itself too much and is taking over, such as Californian poppies (*Eschscholzia californica*). Some 'weeds', such as teasel, make beautiful, statuesque plants, whose thistly tops are loved by birds for winter food. They are as tough as old boots with one long, fat tap root that once established is a pig to dislodge. If left to self-seed, teasels will quickly muscle out many more sensitive plants, but if strictly rationed with a sprinkling of them around the garden, they bring a carefree, naturalistic feel to a place. Like sensible use of salt in a meal, they can be just what a garden needs.

Keeping weeds at bay, in an organic system, is more labour-intensive than the cop-out of using chemicals, but you can reduce the amount of work required in any given area by not letting weeds get out of hand in the first place. Once you have cleared an area, it is straightforward enough to keep on top of the problem with regular hoeing. A hoe is designed for dispatching young weeds as well as breaking up earth at the surface of the soil. Push it into the earth no more than a couple of centimetres deep to dislodge young weed seedlings, then remove them or leave them to rot on the soil surface.

This is the treatment for annual, self-sown seedlings – usually the easiest to deal with. Such weeds have the irritating habit of being very successful plants, capable of producing several generations in one season. But catch them before they flower and you have a chance of getting the upper hand.

Perennial weeds are a greater problem because once established, they come back year after year. If you chop off the top of a perennial with the hoe, leaving some of it behind in the soil, it will likely grow back. Common weeds in this category include the dandelion, dock and plantain with long, thin 'tap' roots that go straight down into the soil. These are best dealt with by digging the root out with a trowel or fork, hoping that no part of them gets left behind.

That autumn term, one of our beds was so full of weeds it looked like we had been deliberately cultivating them. So thick were they in parts that they threatened to overwhelm the leeks with which they shared space – and leeks, as any gardener knows, are no pushover. One of the reasons we had so many interlopers, I suspect, was not entirely down to neglect. A substantial part of one of the raised beds consisted of home-made compost that had been given to us by someone in the village, and I had a theory that it had come with dormant seedlings in there, or perhaps some chunks of dock root, which were particularly thick on this bit of ground.

With such enthusiasm for weeding on tap, a few sessions of the term were spent clearing the worst of the beds. We would be planting garlic, cabbage, onions and, oh yes, more broad beans before we broke up for the year, and they needed somewhere to go.

Where there were still French beans, sweet peas and the tattered remains of red cabbage and sprouts to provide competition, the weeds had made less of an impact. We decided to clear only the areas of weeds that threatened to go to seed and make matters worse: the remaining intruders could stay for the winter, where they would act as ground cover until we could do something about them in the spring.

Disposing of your weeds is not as simple as throwing them on the compost to rot down. Those dandelion clocks that you have carefully removed from your borders so that no seeds are left behind could grow or remain dormant in the compost if that is where you put them. A compost heap can get very hot and kill off the seeds, but it's a gamble. The same goes for perennial roots. Only really hot composting guarantees that everything is safely disposed of.

As a rule, annual weeds can be composted if they have not seeded. Perennial leaves are OK, too. Perennial roots, however, should be bagged up like autumn leaves and left to decay over time.

Compost

Composting is one of those gardening jobs traditionally sorted out in the autumn when you are supposed to be less busy, though topping up and maintaining a compost heap is year-round. At the school, there are three compost bins at the back of the polytunnel, two of the common, dalek-shaped variety and another more box-shaped one. Kitchen peelings and break-time fruit are collected then emptied into one of these larger bins by the children. The bins also contain leaves, twigs and the occasional sweet or crisp wrapper.

According to the government-backed recycling campaign, RecycleNow, 34 per cent of British gardeners now practise some form of home composting. This is regarded as a positive figure, but strikes me as alarming, given that it's such an easy thing to do. It is not as if composting is demanding: it's not like recycling tin cans, which have to be washed, or remembering to take old carrier bags to the supermarket. You just have to chuck it all in a heap in the corner of the garden.

Composting is important in fighting global warming, too. According to WRAP, waste reduction and recycling advisers to the government, when organic matter is sent to landfill, it gets trapped under other waste and decomposes without oxygen. This results in the production of methane, a powerful greenhouse gas. When it breaks down in a compost bin, no methane is produced, which is good news for the environment.

Composting is an integral part of the gardening process, not only giving you a useful place to put all your garden debris, but providing top quality, free food for your soil and plants in years to come. Whole books are written on the subject and it is easy to become a compost obsessive, but the basic rules of composting are straightforward. Follow these and you'll soon get a feel for what you are doing right and wrong. Here are some key pointers for getting a compost heap right.

For successful compost you need air, warmth, water and lots of worms and micro-organisms to break it all down. One of the main reasons compost heaps or bins go wrong is because they have too much of one thing, be it grass cuttings or kitchen waste. Think of it like a balanced diet: apples are good for you, but how would you fare if apples were all you ate? You should aim for a mix of all sorts of gardening ingredients, so if, for example, you have large amounts of grass cuttings that are going into the pile and little else, the heap will not be successful. Best to put most of those cuttings in a separate pile, or use as a mulch, so there is more of a balance between kitchen waste and plant material.

A compost heap should not be too wet, not too dry. In a very hot summer, it might benefit from the occasional bucket of water. When it is looks like it is getting too soggy, put in some shredded newspaper, straw or cardboard.

Some things to avoid or use sparingly:

Leaves (see below)

Twigs, like leaves, will not break down as quickly as other garden waste. You are probably OK with small amounts of woody stems such as roses, but on the whole, twigs should be shredded (not very feasible at a gardening club) or put in a separate pile. They will eventually break down and meanwhile can be a home for hibernating insects.

Cooked food should not be added to the heap, unless you want to attract rats.

Uncooked meat, fish and dairy produce, though crushed eggshells don't seem to present a problem.

Perennial weeds Unless you manage to get a very hot heap, these could survive the composting process. Best to put dandelions, dock and other persistent perennials in a bucket of water, let them rot thoroughly and then add them to the heap.

Grass cuttings make for a great 'activator' of compost, but should be used sparingly to stop your heap turning into a slushy mess. Grass clippings are a great mulch, which can be put around the base of beans to prevent moisture loss in hot weather.

Citrus fruit peel will kill off worms in a compost heap if too much is added.

Open versus 'closed' heap

A compost heap benefits from being regularly 'turned', especially in summer when it is at its warmest and most active. This will bring in oxygen and help decomposition. Turning a heap is, in principle, simple: stick a garden fork into it and turn it over, moving the stuff on the bottom to the top. But it is easier said than done. If you have a dalek-style bin, you could empty it on to a sheet of tarpaulin; the children and you could then go through it, seeing what rots more quickly than the rest, before returning it to the bin. Ideally, you'd have an empty dalek bin to turn the contents of the full one into. Some compost anoraks also recommend drilling holes in the sides of the bin, towards the bottom, so that air can get in.

If you are poking around in the compost with a fork, poke carefully. In summer, slowworms might be nesting in its warmth, while from autumn onwards creatures such as hedgehogs could be hibernating in there. This is a good argument for leaving well alone at this time of year, when the benefits of turning the heap are fewer.

Compost bins have their advantages, even if turning the compost in them is going to be difficult. The fact that they are enclosed helps to keep the compost warm, while the lid helps to prevent it becoming saturated in the rain. If you have an open heap, covering the top with an old carpet will really make a difference.

Composting tricks

If there seems to be little action in the heap (most likely it will look like a soggy mess), nettles and comfrey are good 'activators' to help get the composting process moving. A shovelful of garden soil also helps.

If your compost bin is deluged by fruit flies, leave the lid off for 24 hours and predators should take care of them. If there are ants, just add water.

Site your bin or compost heap on bare earth: it will drain better and be accessed more easily by organisms that help the composting process.

Your compost is ready to use when it is dark, dry and crumbly. Enjoy.

Composting in a small space

You don't need a huge amount of space to make good compost, and a compact alternative is a worm bin. Worm bins take up little room and provide an excellent alternative, so long as you aren't of a squeamish disposition – and can afford one.

If you have a worm bin, don't add citrus fruit peel and remember, those worms are pets of a sort: they are relying on you for their food, so what will you do over the long holiday?

Bokashi bins are similar to wormeries in that they don't take up much room and have no odour. You can feed them just about anything from the kitchen, including meat, fish and cooked food. To recycle with a bokashi bin, you must add layers of bokashi 'bran' in between layers of waste. This bran is a complex mixture that includes wheat bran and bacteria, which breaks down waste with a fermentation process rather than putrefication – hence the lack of smell. The bin has a tap at the bottom, from which you extract bokashi juice which, diluted, makes excellent plant food.

Note: a bokashi and a worm bin are designed for kitchen waste as opposed to large amounts of green waste from the garden.

In an ideal world, you should have three compost areas or bins: one for this year, one for last year, and the one you made

project

Make your own potting compost

Garden compost on its own is a lovely thing, but is far too concentrated to use as a potting compost. You can make your own, however, by mixing up equal parts of homemade compost, ordinary soil and sharp sand (cheaper from a builder's merchant than from a garden centre). Why not try growing the same seeds in your own compost and compost bought from the garden centre. Are there any differences in the results?

the year before that is now ready to use. If that world really was perfect, you would label each bin, one with a 'use this' and two with the previous years' dates on them. Even better, the current year's bin could have a list of what and what not to put in it.

Suppliers and support: most local authorities supply discount compost bins; contact your council's recycling officer. For a range of worm composting products, try Wiggly Wigglers (0800 216990, wigglywigglers.co.uk). For composting courses and advice sheets, contact the HDRA (024 7630 3517, hdra.org.uk). Government information is at recyclenow.com.

Leaf mould

Leaf mould is the remains of decayed leaves, and is a dark brown friable material not unlike normal garden compost. Leaves are best composted separately because they take longer to decompose: this is because they are broken down by the slower action of fungi, as opposed to the bacteria that more speedily decays most other compost ingredients. A decent leaf mould will mostly consist of deciduous leaves: pine needles and evergreen leaves should be used very sparingly.

A common way to compost leaves is to make a cage from a length of wire mesh: take a piece about 1.5m long, then join the ends together using bits of wire to make a cylinder. One open end sits on the ground, and into the other you feed the leaves. Over time, the heap will rot down to give you an excellent soil improver.

Alternatively, gather leaves up in bin bags, or old compost bags, then seal them at the top, put them out of the way in a corner of the garden and forget about them. Make sure you puncture a few holes in the bags to let air in or the composting process will not work. After a couple of years, you should have lovely leaf mould for the garden.

Mulching

The most sensible way to keep an area clear of weeds is to plant it and I should have thought about doing this for the summer holidays. Leaving land unused will not only expose it to more aggressive colonisers but it will damage its fertility as the weather causes nutrients to leach away. Planting it, on the other hand, will provide competition for any unwanted seeds lurking in the ground. This is the principle behind green manure in the veg patch and so-called ground cover – a planting of tough, low, often evergreen species such as periwinkle that smother the competition and keep an area virtually maintenance free.

But going for such a minimum maintenance option, the sort of thing you find in public parks and outside office blocks, surely goes against the idea of an active gardening club? You want to use your ground, not fix it so that you can all put your feet up. In which case, if there is ever going to be a time when parts of your garden are left unplanted, you should go for some other kind of mulch.

A mulch is something you use to cover the soil's surface and can be anything from 'organic' mulch, meaning something that breaks down, such as plants and bark chippings, to inorganic, such as plastic sheeting and ground glass. Mulch has several advantages. Firstly, it locks moisture into the ground, helping the plants growing in it to get through dry periods. Secondly, organic mulches, such as manure, add nutrients to the soil. A mulch also insulates the soil and whatever is in it against temperature extremes. And it can, depending on the sort of mulch you use, prevent weeds growing.

You have probably seen allotments where whole patches of earth have been covered in black plastic sheeting. This is to kill off weeds underneath by depriving them of light, and keep others out until the growers get round to planting it. Old compost bags can be used instead of sheeting, which is a bit more environmentally sound because at least you are recycling the plastic. Although this is a popular organic means of weed control, the plastic might have to be left on the ground for up to 18 months depending on what monsters you are trying to kill off. Also, a long spell under plastic could be a problem for the ground underneath, affecting the aeration of the soil and the beneficial life that is in there. It might also be keeping slugs warm and giving them a hiding place – out of the sunshine and out of your sight.

Mulching is often done in early spring, to lock moisture into the soil and before the weeds have got going. But if you have a clear patch of ground in early autumn that you do not intend to plant until the following spring, you could sow a 'green manure' that will act not only as a mulch but as a fertiliser, too. Green manures are fast-maturing plants such as clover, winter field beans and white mustard that, typically, are dug into the ground before a new crop is planted. Not only do they slow down soil erosion while growing, but they also prevent nutrients being leached out of the soil by rain. When the plants are dug into the ground before a new 'real' crop is planted, they are in effect a compost material. If your green manure is a leguminous plant, it will 'fix' beneficial nitrogen into the soil, too. (Remember if using such plants to bear in mind crop rotation in your garden: *see page 61*.) No wonder organic gardeners swear by the stuff.

A green manure can be any plant grown for this purpose, but plants typically sold under this banner include clovers, beans and peas and mustard. Green manures to sow in early autumn include vetches and grazing rye or rye grass. In school, once we had finished our autumn planting, we sowed mustard on any remaining patches of bare earth. This was great fun for the children, breaking all the rules of seed sowing by sprinkling whole handfuls of the stuff on the ground. Strictly speaking, however, mustard is not an ideal green manure to sow at this time of year, because it will not get through a harsh winter. But it just happened to be the green manure that I had at home so we thought we would give it a go. It came up in no time, and survived the winter, which says more about the mildness of the weather than my horticultural know-how.

Another environmentally friendly mulch that can be used instead of plastic to kill off weeds is cardboard. It is best applied in three or more layers, soaked with water to help hold it down, then piled up with another organic matter such as compost (thus serving the double purpose of concealing a soggy eyesore but creating fertile growing medium for the spring). Cardboard is free and you can get the children to bring it into school; they will love wetting it and putting it round the plants: I'll leave you to work out the details. When the time comes to plant, you can either dig it into the ground where it will decompose, or cut holes in the cardboard and plant straight though it.

Pruning: the basics

Pruning is one of those gardening topics that can get incredibly complicated, and full marks to anyone who has the staying power to read, let alone write, one of the many books that are devoted to the subject. However, there are some basic rules about pruning and cutting back plants that are useful to know. Combine these with the pruning instructions on the plant label – or in the absence of a label, the specifics you have looked up – and you should have sufficient expertise to get the best from your plants.

One thing about pruning we have learned at gardening club is that it is boring if you are watching. This became painfully apparent when I decided to demonstrate how to restore a climbing rose that had got leggy from neglect. I am sure the turnout dropped the following week.

The advantages of pruning can be difficult to show in the

short term; it doesn't look convincing to the inexperienced eye if you are cutting a dormant rose to a fraction of its former self, or reducing a mass of buddleia to a few centimetres from the ground. You might well say, 'Come back in a few months and you will see why this was the right thing to do.' But when your audience is made up of children unused to the idea of long-term solutions, this is not likely to go down well.

There are several reasons for pruning. Firstly, pruning can help to maintain healthy growth and vigour. You might also want to reduce a plant's size, for cosmetic reasons or because it has outgrown its space. The correct pruning of certain plants helps to promote flowering and fruiting.

Always try to have clean and sharp cutting tools. Dirty tools might be harbouring diseases that you will spread to other plants when you prune them. Sharp tools are necessary to make a clean cut, lessening the chance of disease or rot getting into the plant.

Begin by removing any dead, damaged or diseased branches. You should make your cut immediately above a bud or a side shoot. This means that there is little branch remaining to die off and become infected, lessening the chance of disease spreading into the living parts of the plant.

Your cut should be made at an angle, so that rain does not collect in the cut, which could put it at risk of rotting. This way, the rain instead runs off the angle harmlessly.

What overall shape should you aim for? Stand back and you will soon see if you are making a pig's ear of your pruning. You do not want the plant to look top-heavy or imbalanced. With most plants, your aim should be to keep the centre open in a goblet shape; this allows air to circulate around the plant, promoting healthy growth and lessening the chances of fungal disease setting in.

A bud will grow in the direction it is facing, so bear this in mind when you are pruning. If you are trying to open out the centre of a shrub, for example, inward-facing buds will simply grow back into the space you have created.

Generally speaking, you should not cut into old wood on evergreens, such as lavender. Lavender and similar southern European shrubs, such as cistus and rosemary, respond to a trim straight after flowering, when you can remove old blooms and shape the plant. If you live in a particularly cold area, however, it is best to wait to do this in the spring.

Some popular shrubs can be pruned hard every year. The elderberry family, buddleia (butterfly bush), caryopteris and perovskia are cut right back in spring to flower later in the year. *Kerria japonica*, with its shock of orangey-yellow flowers early in the season, is a boring green blob for the rest of the year. This is one worth chopping right back straight after flowering, to allow other plants the space.

Roses respond to hard pruning, too, although this requires a certain exactness. There is a saying that you should let your enemy prune your roses, because if you do it yourself you might not be sufficiently ruthless. Correct pruning of roses, however, will bring rewards in the form of better-looking plants and more flowers.

Bush roses can be pruned by about one third at the end of the year, so they are less likely to get damaged by the winter winds. In spring you should prune them again, cutting back to healthy buds – and I mean right back – while trying to maintain a goblet shape. Remove old and dead stems at the base.

Climbing and rambler roses can be encouraged to flower by training the stems towards the horizontal. This will encourage side shoots to form, which will flower. Cut out old, dark brown branches at their base.

But before you prune any plant, it is best to look it up in a book such as *How to Prune* by John Cushnie. Your gardening club might have some fruit trees, for example, and they will have particular needs if you want them to fruit properly the following season.

Fame at last

Although experienced gardeners would have been appalled by our weed situation – come to think of it, anyone would: it looked a mess – I felt that our garden was finally coming together. The raised beds looked like a genuine veg patch that you could raid for the kitchen. The French beans – the very same ones that in August brought us glory at the village show – had been served for school lunch, though they were increasingly stringy as the crop became too mature. There was a thriving parsley patch, too, desperately in need of harvesting if only we could find someone to take it off our hands. We gave loads of it to the village shop, but it didn't seem to make a difference.

Another indication that we had gelled as a gardening club was the attention we were getting outside the school.

The horticultural society was keen to help. I got a phone call out of the blue to say that they had just had their annual general meeting and called in subscriptions. They wanted to give us some money to spend on anything we liked. Would £100 do? Thank you, horticultural society; sorry I was a bit rude about your show.

There was also attention from further afield. Towards the end of the summer term, I had been asked to meet one of the organisers of *Screen Bites*, the Dorset festival of film and food that takes place every autumn. *Screen Bites* wanted to know whether the gardening club could be involved, possibly supplying the kitchen for a visit by the renowned local chef Ian Simpson, proprietor of the White House in Charmouth, who would cook lunch for the children. The results would be filmed and shown as part of the festival.

While it was flattering to think that our veg could be touched by the hand of an award-winning chef, I was nonetheless reluctant to guarantee him any produce. We were still feeling our way and, when I met up with the *Screen Bites* people, I had no idea what would survive the summer holidays into autumn. Perhaps with a little more experience, I would have felt more confident. As it turned out, the wet summer meant he could have had our French beans in September.

There was another offer from *Screen Bites*, however, that was far more tempting. The local garden centre was sponsoring the festival and keen to support schools growing their own food. Would I be interested in talking to them?

Of course I was. The gardening club resources were not exactly buoyant. More like rock bottom. The school had promised to reimburse me for day-to-day expenses – seeds, plants and compost – whenever I got around to sending in my receipts, but there had been no mention of anything beyond that. The garden centre could mean bigger things – in the business world they would call it infrastructure.

We had a few functioning tools, but the majority were not child-friendly, being too large and unwieldy for a small person. Compost was always in short supply and though it was full of plants, the polytunnel had an unloved feel about it. We were down to one decent watering can and every Tuesday before our sessions I traipsed grumpily around the school, looking for the one remaining rose that fitted it. Why did the roses always disappear? What did the children find to do with them? The only other decent watering can now had a big dent in one side and leaked.

Prompted by *Screen Bites*, I sent the garden centre a wishlist for new tools, workbenches for the polytunnel and wood and earth for more raised beds. I talked with the children about what they might like, equipment-wise, and foam kneelers were a real favourite. No harm in asking the garden centre for as much as possible, I thought, and was half-expecting a polite 'No' to most of my list, with maybe a watering can or two and some seeds as consolation. But I was wrong – they said yes to everything.

The tools and accessories you will need for a gardening club might differ slightly from those usually used. As for how many of each to get, ultimately you have to be the judge. I found that we needed more watering cans than I expected (I calculated six for a club whose numbers rarely exceeded a dozen, and with the children watering in pairs). It is a good idea to have enough hand forks and trowels to go round everyone; as for the larger tools, the children seemed happy sharing.

Essential tools for a gardening club

Small watering cans: These are easier for the children to manage. Plastic ones are more practical because they are lighter to carry and cheaper to replace when they inevitably go missing. On the side of each you should write the following request in indelible ink and in large letters: *Please Return to the Gardening Club*. This could be followed by an optional warning containing threats that are likely to deter the cans being borrowed at all, but that could bring you into conflict with the school authorities.

Ideally, each watering can should come with a rose attached to it by a sturdy chain, though I have yet to come across anybody who sells such a combination. If you are similarly unlucky in your search for one, make sure you have a private supply of roses that you bring with you each week, replacing ones that go missing as necessary. A fine rose is best for watering young plants (think of a flour sieve as opposed to a colander).

They can get clogged up with dirt from time to time, but in my experience they are the best way to ensure baby plants have a drink as opposed to a life-threatening dousing.

Hand forks and hand trowels: Be wary of tools that come in sweetshop colours to make them more attractive to children. Some of these are as much use as a credit card on a desert island. It is important that all tools are good quality – even young children can break poor-quality tools in unyielding earth. The sign of a strong trowel is one with a concave blade and a curved handle.

Small spade: Often described as a 'border' or 'lady's' spade in the garden centre, but if such old-fashioned notions irritate you, you can find smaller good-quality tools online; try www.harrodhorticultural.com).

Garden fork: See spade, above.

Rakes: A general-purpose rake will suffice, though it is really worth giving a safety lesson when this tool comes out. We have had our Tom and Jerry moments at school, where a rake with the tines facing upwards has been trodden on and the handle has shot up and bashed a child. A springbok rake is good for raking up grass and leaves, but not much use on bare earth.

Hoe: An essential weeding tool for an adult, though it should be supervised if being used by a child. A Dutch hoe, which you use with a gentle push and pull motion to uproot annual weeds and break up the ground, is as good as any.

Secateurs: One quality pair, always carried by you and never let out of your sight. Price is always a good indication of what you're getting.

Kneeling mats: 'Over-accessorising' I used to think, until our gardening club was given some. This was an epiphany – they do so much to keep children's clothes clean, as well as making weeding more comfortable for your knees. They are cheap and widely available – buy some with bright patterns or flowers printed on them rather than the typical dour utilitarian green.

Child-sized gloves: There will always be common weeds that sting, prick and spike you, but less obvious are the plants that can cause irritation to the skin. A pair of gloves might also encourage a squeamish child to overcome, say, their fear of worms (not a useful phobia to have in a gardening club). Either encourage the children to bring their own gloves, or buy a variety of sizes but in exactly the same design. Otherwise you risk the sort of problem you get in a cafe with different-coloured drinking straws: a choice will only cause arguments.

A notebook: To compare what you did year after year. This will help you to hone your technique with certain plants and learn from your mistakes.

A wheelbarrow or gardener's bag: For gathering weeds. Saves you clearing up.

You might also throw in a riddle for sieving soil (a riddle is a large sieve: I always brought my own to school) and a soil thermometer, which might be the key to an interesting project or two. And, at the risk of stating the obvious, a new gardening club will have to have a good supply of the following: garden canes (more than you think you will need and in varying sizes: those 8ft ones in the garden centre are worth it if you're going to grow beans); gardening twine; large plastic pots (10cm and 20cm) for potting on, and seed trays and modules for getting your plants going. Modules are the trays that are divided up like egg cartons into individual parts. The idea is that each module, or cell, has its own plant in it and the benefits are reduced competition from other seedlings, and less chance of trauma for the plant when it is transplanted. This is because the module can be moved in its entirety, with the roots encased in their own private bit of compost.

The *Screen Bites* day arrived, and a reinvigorated gardening club was there to meet the PR people, a camera crew and the local paper. The older children in the group were allowed out of classes for the occasion and we were all photographed and filmed sowing broad beans, and planting onion bulbs (called sets) and baby spring cabbage that had been brought in by the garden centre. I have moaned about cabbage grown in the spring, but this was different. For one, it was free. Secondly, it was less prone to pests this time of year and would be ready the following spring, giving us something to harvest early in the season.

We had our few minutes of fame in a food documentary shown at the festival and in community centres around the county. On screen the children talked of the magic of growing food – articulate ambassadors for our modest little set-up.

Into winter

There was plenty to do throughout autumn at gardening club and because of a few cancellations due to bad weather, what I had expected to run until half term at the end of October actually went on until late the following month. By then, the children were well into their preparations for the carol service and other Christmas events, and gardening club was getting in the way. Numbers had been dwindling, too, mirroring the decline of the garden, and a couple of times only three or four of us turned up.

Over the term, tasks included clearing the meadow, sowing sweet peas and purslane indoors, potting up strawberry runners and, as always when there was a spare moment, weeding the beds. By the last day, despite the stop-start run we had had of late, we went out with a bang rather than a stutter. Seven children turned up – good considering recent attendance – including a couple of new faces. It was a damp, murky day, but also very mild, so we potted up some more strawberry runners that I had planned to compost (no harm in trying), sowed green manure on a spare patch of soil and got our garlic in, too.

There are two things I like about garlic besides the flavour. Firstly, I have always found it easy to grow, and secondly it is something you can plant in late autumn, just when you thought there was nothing else to do in the garden. It is one of the better things to plant with children, who enjoy breaking up the garlic bulbs, making nice fat holes with a dibber or handle of a trowel, and popping a clove into each one. It made a suitable finale to the end of the gardening club year.

What of the future? There would be much to do the following term, but I had agreed with the head teacher that we would start after half term. This was to give me time to construct four new raised beds, narrower this time, that our friendly garden centre had promised us, and I hoped these would encourage the rest of the school to get more involved in the garden. The idea was to give each of the four classes in the school (which, it being a small establishment, covered the entire age range) responsibility for one of these new beds, and hopefully bring gardening into curriculum time. A big frustration for me had been getting the remainder of the school to become involved in the garden, rather than it all depending on a volunteer and the children's willingness to turn up in their lunch hour. The excuse was always that the curriculum was busy enough, but other primary schools managed to do this, so why not us?

With new beds in place, more tools and the experience of gardening club veterans, surely this was enough to start a green-fingered revolution. The children and their teachers would be able to plant what they liked in these new beds; they wouldn't have to fit in with what gardening club did on a Tuesday lunchtime. Just so long as they didn't upstage us.

We had also been contacted by the local senior school, to see if there were any one-off projects some of their students could be involved in. They would help us build the new beds and, maybe, an expanded compost area. It should be fun transferring the existing half-rotten compost to its new home, then we could re-site the plastic bins near the kitchen so in wet weather no one would be expected to traipse across the sodden turf.

But I wasn't the only one looking forward to the new gardening year. One Monday in early January, two girls ran up to me and asked me if there was gardening club the next day. No, I told them, we would start again after half term. 'Aww,' they chorused, genuine disappointment on their faces. Sad for them, maybe, but it made my day.

End of term report

While I would never have had it any other way, there are many things I have learned from my year and a bit with the gardening club. Here are my hard-won key principles to approach a gardening club and make it a success.

1. Holidays

Plan to plant and crop things in term time. This sounds obvious, yet I have come across venerable organisations offering support to schools who disregard the fact that children are not around for much of the summer. Gardening around the term-time calendar takes a bit of planning. Many flowering plants will come into their own in the middle of the summer holidays, which is a shame because there will be no one there to enjoy them. This is also true for some vegetables: what's the point of sowing, watering, feeding and nurturing a plant, only to leave it to rot or turn into something tough and inedible while you are on vacation? Having said all this, rules are there to be broken: we do grow some things, such as tomatoes or pumpkins in pots. The children can take them home with them and grow them during the summer holiday.

2. Make it easy on yourself

The children come to gardening club in order to plant things and watch them grow. It is sensible to assume, then, that their interest might start to waver if, say, a tray of seeds fail to germinate. Such little setbacks and dramas can happen to any gardener, but why put yourself under such pressure? Surely it is better to cultivate reliable plants such as broad beans, or bulbs that anyone with a modicum of commonsense can, in a matter of months, turn into lusty plants.

If anything is slightly tricky – carrots are a good example, being notoriously difficult to grow on our heavy soil – why put yourself through the pain of growing them? It is surely best for everyone that what you sow or plant comes up and delivers what it says on the pack.

Don't be too proud to buy baby 'plug' plants, either, if decent ones come your way. It is more expensive to do this, but I'm assuming you don't have a couple of acres to fill up, so we're talking a few extra pounds every now and then. In terms of satisfaction for the children, and humiliation spared on your part, it is a sound investment. But really, stay away from the difficult stuff. The children have got their whole lives before them: the bonsai and bananas can come later.

3. Food factor

When I started the gardening club, I wanted more than an ornamental garden and I guessed that growing things to eat would appeal to the children, too. So far, this has proved to be right, so there is an emphasis on growing food. We aim to grow vegetables that the children like to eat, but not at the expense of our self-esteem. Therefore we sometimes end up growing things that the children might not like to eat, such as rocket. This can always be taken home for the family, so everyone is happy in the end.

4. From Turkey Twizzlers to tasty veg

Jamie Oliver was famously appalled at the processed Turkey Twizzlers being served at a school he worked with – his point being children should be eating better quality, healthier food for their lunch.

If your school has an in-house kitchen, grow things that can be included on the menu and the children can try at mealtimes. This makes it more fun for them, and introduces the idea of healthy eating by the back door, instead of snooze-inducing lectures on the subject. Potatoes are an obvious example of something that is reasonably easy to grow (with the odd exception such as our first summer) and liked by a lot of children. We had a lot of success with salad, too.

5. Size matters

A small child is never going to be able to lug around a normal-sized watering can, nor usefully wield an adult spade or fork – this might even be questionable from a health and safety point of view. It is important, then, that the children have access to tools that fit them, so they are not frustrated when trying to do normal gardening tasks.

6. The only way is up

If in doubt about your soil, or if you only have concrete outside space, then build raised beds. These will provide you with an instant garden without any of the grief of trying to work with the earth you've got. Alternatively, try planting in containers – there are few limits on what you can grow, as long as you can find a container big enough. Be aware though that soil in containers dries out quickly and plants in containers need to be kept watered more than those in the ground. They also benefit from feeding.

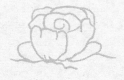

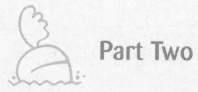

Part Two

week by week through the seasons

We started our gardening club in the summer term, but a good time to begin the school gardening year is after the spring half-term holiday, which usually falls at the end of February. Look through the following pages in advance and try to order seed you'll want for the whole season. Unfortunately, it is not as easy as popping down to the garden centre – even the best won't have all the varieties you want to grow – and using the best seed for your local conditions could be the difference between success and failure.

sPring term

WEEK ONE

Sow beetroot

Children should enjoy growing beetroot if only because it is such a pretty plant. Perhaps they can be persuaded to try eating it, too: beetroot eaten as a young root, boiled or roasted, is a totally different experience from eating fibrous old bruisers or slimy mass-produced pickles that might have traumatised a young palate. And young beetroot, picked before the summer holidays, when it is the size of a ping-pong ball, is what you are after here.

Beetroot is one of those plants that does not like being transplanted, but you can get round this by sowing it in individual modules, which have more room for the roots and can be transplanted lock, stock and barrel. As an alternative to modules, get the children to bring in old yoghurt pots, make a few drainage holes in the bottom of them with the end of a knife or fork, and sow into these.

First, soak the seeds overnight, then sow 2cm deep, and try to have just one seed per module, which might mean supervising each child to make sure the seeds end up where they are supposed to go. Beetroot seeds are a good size and easy to handle so sowing this way should not be difficult – anyhow, don't panic if more than one seed ends up in the module. The children will want to write their names on the pots, but I try to discourage this: what if little Emma's seed doesn't germinate and the rest do?

Most beet seeds are actually a cluster of seed, so several 'seedlings' should appear in each module. These can be left as they are and will form a clump of small beets later in the season. When seedlings are 5cm high, plant out the modules, spacing them about 20cm apart each way.

Which varieties to grow?

This is early to be planting beetroot, which could bolt (go to flower) before you get a decent-sized root. But needs must: you want to crop your beets before the end of next term, and though you are after small roots because they are tastier, you don't want them to be diddy. The beetroot you should sow around this time of year, therefore, need to be bolt-resistant varieties. Boltardy and Pronto fit the bill perfectly.

To harvest, pull out the roots when they are needed, then twist off the leaves. If the children are not wearing old clothes, they should be careful when handling the beets because their juice will stain. Wear gloves also, ideally a set of rubber ones shared between you, to stop the juice staining hands.

Beetroot is an easy vegetable to cultivate with few problems, but birds can be a pest. When you plant them out, get the children to rig up a deterrent using cotton and sticks: find some sturdy sticks or bamboo canes at least 30cm long, four for each row; push two of the sticks into the ground at the end of each row, about 10cm apart so they form a rectangle that encloses the row. Now tie six lengths of cotton, about 10cm off the ground, between the sticks in each row: this way, if one length breaks the whole thing will not unravel. You should now have a box shape with a diagonal X inside it for each row which will help prevent birds landing and eating the plants.

Finally, if the ground gets too dry while the beetroot is growing, the roots can become woody. If there is then a sudden burst of rain, this can cause splitting. To get around this, keep the beetroot watered. No problems there, I imagine.

PROS

- One of the easiest vegetables to grow.
- Largely disease-free.
- Its pretty leaves look good anywhere in the garden.
- Delicious when eaten young.

CONS

- Will need to be started indoors this early in the season.
- Can be slow to germinate.
- Children might take some persuading to eat it.
- Beetroot sown early are prone to bolting so it is important you buy a 'bolt-resistant' variety.
- Beets can get fibrous if soil is allowed to dry out.
- Needs protecting from birds.

Don't forget ...

- Did you overwinter any salad in the polytunnel or greenhouse? Can it be cut now?
- How are your autumn-sown broad beans looking? Do they need supporting?
- Did you sow winter bedding in your containers? How is it looking? Do you need to clear it now and let the spring bulbs through?
- Order seed potatoes or go out and buy them now: it is already getting late and you might not be guaranteed the variety you want. You don't want to be left with everyone else's rejects at the garden centre.
- Sweet peas can still be sown indoors, though flowering might be later than those sown last autumn.
- Have you ordered all the other seeds you want for this season? If not, get on the phone to your chosen supplier.
- Begin sowing leeks from any time now.

Pollution and your garden

If your garden is near a main road, consider plants that are tolerant of pollution. These include buddleia, ceanothus, forsythia, lilac, mock orange.

If you are worried about pollution on your vegetables, most pollutants, including pesticides, lead and fungicides remain in the outer skin, so always peel your root veg.

WEEK TWO

Sow tomatoes

In a good summer, certain varieties of tomato can be grown outdoors but are unlikely to crop before the summer holidays. One solution is to get an earlier crop by growing them indoors (in a greenhouse or polytunnel or on a sunny windowledge) either in a container or growbags designed specifically for tomatoes. The latter are ideal because you won't have to worry about feeding plants at a later stage: lie the bag on the ground and plant tomatoes through holes cut in the top. If you grow the tomatoes in a container, however, the children can take plants home at any stage of the summer, and it does not matter if they have not cropped before the end of the term.

Seed should be started off inside. If you have a heated greenhouse, you could sow as early as December, but this is getting really technical and, I think, decadent in these times of climate change. For a school gardening club attempting an indoor crop by July, the ideal time to sow seed would be in the last week of February, or early March.

If you are prepared to wait until the following term for your tomato plants, an alternative is to buy or scrounge some seedlings. Typically at the end of April and into May, there are plenty of cheap baby plants in the garden centres or being sold with an honesty box at the end of driveways. Other green-fingered parents might want to donate some to the school – or a local garden centre might be encouraged to do so. In our school, the village horticultural society annually donates a young tomato plant to every child in the school, asking them to grow them on at home and enter them in the village show in August. But really, tomato seeds are generally easy to grow and by sowing your own you'll get more choice of variety.

Tomatoes can either be sown in seed trays 2cm deep, then pricked out when they are large enough, or grown individually in modules or 9cm pots (best to sow two seeds in each pot, and later thin out the weaker seedling). Tomato seeds are surprisingly tough, so don't give up on their germination: we've had seedlings struggle through despite regular flooding from over-enthusiastic watering.

Keep the compost moist rather than wet, and if starting them in a tray, pot on to 9cm pots when the seedlings have two leaves. Eventually, they should be potted on to a container at least 23cm across – do this at the end of April/early May if growing on indoors, later if they are to go outdoors.

Tomatoes grown on the window ledge, or in a greenhouse or polytunnel, tend to be cordon varieties (one single stem). They should be supported with a cane, or string suspended from the top of the polytunnel or greenhouse. When tying up the plant, leave enough room for the stem to thicken. As your tomatoes grow, remove any growth at the base as well as the small shoots that appear at a 45-degree angle between the stem and the main horizontal branches. The maintenance of tomatoes is labour-intensive, but for a gardening club this should be seen as a positive thing: the children enjoy it, racing each other to find shoots that need to be removed, more of which will appear by the next week's get-together. And their ongoing contact with their tomatoes – as opposed to a less demanding crop – will have a direct bearing on the health of the plants and the quality of the end product.

Your plants will need stopping at some point to prevent them putting on more growth and instead concentrate on building and ripening the fruit. This is typically when an indoor variety reaches the top of the greenhouse or polytunnel (nowhere for the plant to go). To stop the plant, remove the growing point a couple of leaves above the topmost truss.

Watering tomatoes is something of an art form, and tasteless, mushy fruit are often blamed on overwatering. Containers should not be allowed to dry out completely, but kept moist rather than saturated. Tomato aficionados reckon that allowing the pot to almost dry out between waterings improves flavour. If you set up a watering rota in the summer term, make sure the children are aware of this.

Tomatoes are greedy and will benefit from a feed as fruit begins to form. The tomato feed on offer at many garden centres often contains artificial chemicals, though you might find one that doesn't (Miracle-gro now has an organic fertiliser, for example). Making your own feed, on the other hand, costs nothing more than the price of a few comfrey plants (*see page 37 on how to make comfrey tea*). To harvest your tomatoes, break off the little stem where it swells, just above the fruit.

Which varieties to grow?

Here you are spoilt for choice, but it depends to some extent what you want to do with your tomatoes. If you sow just one batch in the gardening club, it would be best to sow varieties that are suited to both indoor and outdoor cultivation. Then you can keep some in the polytunnel or on a sunny classroom window ledge to crop before the end of the summer term. The remainder can be sent home with the children, where they can continue to be grown outside if necessary. Moneymaker and Alicante, both traditional stalwarts of the amateur grower, are suitable for this purpose, the latter with a much superior flavour. Small Fry is another. My absolute favourite, however, has to be the cherry-type Gardener's Delight – a reliable, heavy cropper that is good indoors or out, and manages a perfect balance between sweetness and acidity. Most importantly, children love it.

If your tomatoes are going to stay indoors, then consider Shirley, another popular variety that is a heavy cropper and has good disease resistance. For something different, Golden Sunrise is a yellow variety and Big Boy a popular beefsteak. Tigerella is easy, tasty and, as the name suggests, has yellow and red stripes. It will not crop as heavily as some of the better known varieties.

If you don't have a polytunnel or greenhouse, you can still grow outdoor tomatoes. They will need to germinate on a sunny windowledge, however, after being sown at the end of March or early April. Pot indoors and then harden off your plants towards the end of May. If you are growing a cordon variety, you could do worse than one of those recommended above, but it will need stopping earlier than if it was grown indoors, to guarantee that the fruit will ripen over the summer. This is usually done after small fruits have started forming on the fourth truss. So-called bush varieties are popular as outdoor tomatoes because they are easier to grow and do not need supporting or trimming. Popular varieties include Totem and Red Alert.

An advantage with outdoor tomatoes is that they are less prone to pests and disease than those grown indoors. The exception is blight, the same disease that affects potatoes, where yellow-brown blotches will appear on the leaves. This is prevalent in late summer if the weather is warm and moist, and growers recommend that tomatoes are not grown near potatoes. If plants are attacked by blight – unlikely earlier in the summer but you never can be sure – remove affected leaves and burn them. If this is not possible, seal them in a bag and chuck them out with the normal rubbish. Never compost them.

The main pests for indoor tomatoes are greenfly and whitefly. You can deter them by companion planting of tagetes, nasturtiums and garlic, which will drive off the creatures with its smell. Biological controls are available for both whitefly and greenfly in the greenhouse (try www.organiccatalog.com).

PROS

- **A good crop for a container.**
- **A plant to take home.**
- **Tomatoes are popular with children.**

CONS

- Take a lot of looking after.
- Pests and diseases to worry about.
- They need to be started indoors.
- If you want a crop before the summer holidays, they will have to be kept indoors.

Don't forget ...

Have you remembered to order Jerusalem artichoke tubers? It's not common for garden centres to stock seed, so you'll have to allow time for some to arrive by post. You can buy tubers form the greengrocer's and use those, but you won't know their quality as plants. Or perhaps, instead, there is a local person who grows them and can spare a few tubers for the school? You won't need many.

Is there a bit of spare grass to turn over to meadow? It is probably time for mowing to begin at school, so ask the head teacher if some of it can stay uncut (see page 75 on how to grow a meadow).

project

Measure out two similar sized areas of land, one where the grass is left to grow and one with cut grass, well away from hedgerows and the long grass. Over the summer term, keep a diary of the insects you spot in each one over the same amount of time – say ten minutes. At the end of term, compare notes. What were the differences?

WEEK THREE

Plant Jerusalem artichokes

It is a mystery to me why more people do not grow Jerusalem artichokes, those knobbly white or pinkish tubers that look a bit like ginger root. Perhaps it is precisely because of their knobbliness, making them a hassle to clean for cooking.

Jerusalem artichokes are one of the easiest and most reliable vegetables to grow, and they are delicious to eat. They have a slightly nutty, sweet flavour and can be eaten raw (sliced for a fresh, crunchy addition to a salad) or cooked – my favourite way is roasting them until the insides collapse into a delicious, creamy mash.

Let's not beat about the bush here: Jerusalem artichokes are supposed to cause flatulence, which perhaps counts against them, but then so do baked beans and sprouts, and you see no shortage of these in the shops. Because of children's unfamiliarity with them, they might be tough to get past the school cook, but you could try (they can always be chopped up in a mince, and help the school kitchen meet fresh vegetable targets set by government). Alternatively, you can sell them at the school gates. They will crop in winter when there is not much interesting fresh produce about, so those parents that know and like Jerusalem artichokes should be queuing up to buy them; those that decline a purchase, well, let them eat sprouts.

Getting started with Jerusalem artichokes is, as with garlic, pricier than most vegetables, because you have to buy the tubers. But also as with garlic, you should look at it as a long-term investment. When you come to harvest them at the end of the year – and make sure you get them all up or they will spread like wildfire – keep back some of the healthiest-looking ones for next year's seed tubers. These should be about the size of an egg with at least two buds on them; large tubers can be cut in half.

Jerusalem artichokes are happy in sun or partial shade and come to that, most soils except ones that get waterlogged. Like potatoes, they are used to break in ground that has not been cultivated and because of their undemanding nature can be put in a corner of the garden that might not suit other plants. Plant them around 15cm deep, 35cm apart and with 90cm between rows.

Jerusalem artichokes are a member of the sunflower family and, like their cousins, can grow very tall, up to 3m. In summer, you should cut them back to at least 2m so they can put energy into developing tubers. At this stage they might also need some support. They are a wonderful plant for children to grow, ticking many of the right boxes (easy, large seed, tall when mature). In late autumn, when their leaves begin to die back, cut down stems to 10cm from the ground and leave your crop where it sits until you are ready to harvest and eat it or sell it. Harvest with a garden fork, gently digging around the roots so as not to damage them but making sure to lift all the tubers.

Which varieties to grow?

There aren't usually that many to choose from. If you can get hold of them, Fusea and the purply-red Gerrard are both smooth-skinned varieties, which will make them easier to clean.

PROS

- Very easy to grow.
- Will tolerate shade.
- Can be grown on difficult ground.
- An interesting fresh veg to harvest in winter when not much else is going on.

CONS

- Will children eat it? Hmm ...
- Can be invasive: leave a tuber in the ground and you'll get another plant.
- Grows large so can shade out other plants if you are not careful.

Don't forget ...

- While potatoes are fresh in your mind, get on the phone and order Christmas potato seeds, to be planted at the end of next term and harvested in winter. Specialists should be taking orders now.
- Are you planning to buy perennial plants for this year? It's an expensive way to garden, but you might have some money for a few treats. Perennials are best planted in the autumn or early spring (typically March) rather than waiting until it is hot and dry, when they might struggle (*more on perennials on page 249*).
- Carrots for cropping in June can be sown from early March.

project

The jam jar soil test

Half fill your jam jar with soil, then fill it up with water. Put the lid on, shake, and leave for a couple of days. The contents should have now settled into layers of particles of different sizes and water. Make sure you can see the different layers. At the bottom there should be large particles, then medium above that, and fine above that. The top of the jar should consist of water with a thin layer of bits floating on top of it – this is organic material.

You can tell whether you have a sandy soil or a clay soil by looking at the largest layer in the jar.

The largest layer of a sandy soil will be the large particles at the bottom of the jar, with thinner layers of medium and fine particles above it.

The largest layer of a clay soil will be the layer of fine particles immediately beneath the water.

WEEK FOUR

Plant potatoes

If you have ever seen potato seed in the garden centre, you will be familiar with the terms 'early' and 'maincrop'. I have always found this slightly off-putting. Such descriptions make the simple spud appear complicated.

A veg garden without potatoes is like pizza without the cheese. It doesn't feel quite right, especially in a school garden where the planting and harvest of potatoes is so tactile and visibly rewarding. And it is a vegetable that even the fussiest child will permit on their plate. Admittedly they do take up a lot of room, but potatoes can be grown in large containers (at least 30 cm deep) or even old compost bags. Allow one seed potato per container, which should only be filled halfway up to allow room for earthing up (see below).

In a nutshell, early and maincrop describe how long the crop takes to reach maturity. Earlies – or new potatoes, which include 'very earlies' and 'second earlies' – come first, in mid summer, and should be eaten straight out of the ground. Maincrop take longer to mature and can be eaten fresh or stored. Earlies take up less space and give you a smaller crop, but they are also harvested when potatoes are at their most expensive, so are the best ones to grow in a small space. If you plant a quick-maturing variety at school, you could supply the kitchen at such inflationary times and save it money. If you have more room, you could plant potatoes for a succession crop, harvesting your new potatoes before the end of the summer term, and leaving the maincrop over the summer for a harvest in September. However, potatoes need water in dry weather, so you are taking a big gamble by leaving any in the ground over the summer holidays. Unless, of course, you can persuade someone to turn up regularly with the watering can.

You can start to plant potatoes in early spring – from mid-March in the south of the country. However, if it is very wet, dry or cold it might be best to wait (perhaps you could sow broad beans this week, instead; *see page 233*). Soil temperature should be around 6°C before planting.

Typically, earlies and second earlies (which crop a few weeks later) go in first, followed by maincrop (mid-April planting, though it can be later if this interferes with the school holidays), the idea being that you will get a succession of spuds over the summer. But you don't have to stick to this timing. All your potatoes can be planted at the same time if you wish.

If you chit potatoes first, you are gaining extra growing time before they go in the earth. This is important if you are after an early crop because you can begin chitting in December and January as seed potato becomes available, but when the ground is too cold to be planted.

Chitting is the process of encouraging the seed potatoes to grow before they go into the earth. The tubers should be put in a cool, light place (out of direct sunlight) and left to sprout shoots. Ideally, the potatoes should be placed on end with their 'rose' end upwards (the end with the most eyes) – old egg boxes are useful to hold them in place. When the shoots are about 2.5cm long, they can go into the ground.

To plant potatoes, dig a trench or individual holes. Early potatoes should be at least 10cm deep, with 30cm between tubers and in rows about 50cm apart; maincrop 15cm deep with 75cm between rows, spacing the potatoes 40cm apart.

As potato shoots emerge, cover them with earth from the ground in between rows, or if they are growing in a container, some more compost. This is known as earthing up and will keep tubers out of the light, preventing them from turning green. Repeat this about once a fortnight and you should end up with ridges about 30cm high with lush green leaves spilling from their tops.

Potatoes are best harvested in dry conditions and left in the open air for an hour or two to dry off. But if you are eager to get them to the cook in time for tomorrow's lunch, they can go straight to the kitchen. Try to dig under the plants with a garden fork to avoid damaging the crop. Earlies are usually ready when the flowers droop and the foliage begins to die back. Maincrop should be left in the ground until needed, though the later you leave it, the more likely the risk of blight (as per tomatoes, see above) and attack by slugs.

Rotation of your crop is important, to avoid other problems with potatoes, notably eelworms. Potatoes are also hungry plants and feeding the ground before planting with either compost, manure, homemade fertiliser such as nettle solution or a green manure will help prevent scab. Scab is a fungal disease that causes unsightly scabby patches on the skin of the potato and is mainly associated with light, dry soils.

Which varieties to grow?

If you are lucky in January and early February, there might be a local potato day in your area. This is where you can get to see and buy a bewildering array of seed spuds and get advice from all manner of potato anoraks. This could be a good place to choose some varieties to grow or the basis for a school trip (the best known event is that held by Ryton Organic Gardens – www. gardenorganic.org.uk – in the Midlands, and there is a potato fair in London at the end of January each year, www.london21.org).

Alternatively, seed catalogues contain extensive selections or you can get advice from one of the school gardening support organisations such as www.potatoesforschools.org.uk.

Potatoes like fertile soil and tolerate many conditions, but some varieties are more suited to particular areas. A good local garden centre should reflect this, or maybe there is a local allotment holder or amateur whose brains you can pick.

Potatoes usually come with advice as to their susceptibility to blight and disease, so to make life easier for yourself go for one that is not going to give you trouble (Kestrel and Winston come recommended among the earlies and Santé as a maincrop). My favourite is the knobbly Pink Fir Apple, a maincrop with exotic looks and earthy taste. When you can find it in the shops, it's expensive, which is all the more reason to grow it. Children might at first be put off by its looks, but once they have tried it and found it to taste like a superior spud, it might give them the confidence to experiment with more exotic unknown food. It is supposedly prone to blight but I have never found this to be the case.

159

PROS

- **Fairly easy to grow.**
- **Children on the whole like to eat them.**
- **A good thing to grow in quantity for the kitchen.**
- **Good for breaking up new ground and won't be too upset by weeds.**

project

If you have a suitable space at school, you could begin chitting some potatoes with the children in early February, as a warm-up to gardening club proper. This would depend on there being somewhere light and cool to store them (you could probably get away with doing this in the polytunnel, providing you don't get a prolonged spell of sunny weather). Alternatively, children could take some seed spuds home in early February, in old egg boxes, then bring them back at the beginning of the following month – they will have to be transported carefully, however, so that their shoots do not break off. Keep some of the same variety back, unchitted, then, at harvest time, you can compare yields.

CONS

- You're going to need a lot of room to grow them year after year: it is very important they are rotated.
- For bumper 'maincrop' yields, you want them to stay in the ground for the summer. But who will water them?
- Blight can be a problem with maincrop.

Don't forget ...

- Pinch out the top 6cm of your autumn-sown broad bean plants when the first pods appear. This helps the plant put more energy into producing pods. It will also help as a blackfly control – the aphids find the tender tips of the broad bean plant particularly enticing.
- Begin harvesting when pods are 6cm long.
- Broad beans can also be sown now, to crop before the end of the summer and extend the season beyond an autumn sowing. With an early spring sowing, however, you increase the risk of an aphid attack in summer.

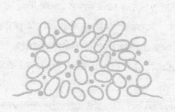

WEEK FIVE

Sow easy summer flowers

What about flowers? By now, the children might be hassling you to grow some, and come to think of it, it's about time you had some blooms to go with your veg. This is a good time to get annuals started, both the hardy and half-hardy versions.

An annual is a plant that takes one season to do its thing. It can be a vegetable or a flower, though gardeners tend to mean the latter when they talk about annuals. You sow seed in the soil, it grows, flowers and dies, all over the course of the year. Annuals are usually sown in March and April, and some will continue pumping out their flowers until late October. With some prolific annuals, such as pot marigolds, there can be more than one generation in a season.

Annuals are perfect to grow with children because you get huge returns in terms of flowers, all from one cheap packet of seed. Some annuals are prolific self-seeders, so you will only need one pack for several years' worth of blooms. Some gardeners find this a nuisance, but if you like a carefree look to your garden, self-seeders will fill in gaps between other flowers and veg. The trick is to recognise what young seedlings look like, to avoid confusing them with weeds. Some, such as California poppies and Love-in-a-mist (*Nigella*), are distinctive as baby plants, so get the children to take a photograph of them as they emerge so you can recognise them for next year.

Hardy annuals can go straight into the ground in late March and early April. You can get an idea of when the soil is warm enough for sowing them because weed seedlings will be appearing. But under a school gardening regime, where you want flowers as soon as possible, it is best to give your annuals a headstart indoors. This also lessens the chance of them being eaten by newly emergent slugs and snails. Our clay soil is wet and cold at this time of year, so save for the toughest of plants (pot marigolds or poached egg plant) or those that really, really hate to be moved (poppies), we sow most annuals indoors and plant them out when they are established.

Half-hardy annuals, such as sunflowers, however, should always be started under cover, then planted out when the risk of frost has

did you know?

Honeybees and bumblebees are extremely important pollinating insects, but not the only bees you are likely to get in the garden. So-called solitary bees include the red mason bee and mining bee and both are also good pollinators. You can encourage these by creating habitats for them: a wooden post with different-sized holes drilled in it, planted in a sunny spot, will make a place for them to lay their eggs, as will the hoverfly hotel on page 212. Bees are attracted to purple, white, yellow and blue flowers, too, but cannot recognise red ones.

passed in May. In warm weather they can be sown straight into open ground, but again are at risk from pests, and are unlikely to perform before the summer holidays. Seed packets should give you a clear indication of the plant's requirements.

Ten easy annuals to grow from seed

Seed companies provide seductive descriptions of thousands of different varieties of annuals, both online and in catalogues, often with an indication of how difficult they are to grow. You and the children could indulge yourselves and go for some unfamiliar faces (in our first year, we grew cladanthus, which has an orange flower like a pot marigold, on top of feathery foliage). However, you can always fall back on some foolproof annuals, such as those listed below, that will fill a garden with colour through the summer. Unless stated otherwise, they are best grown in a sunny site.

California poppy (Eschscholzia) Fine fern-like foliage with orange and sometimes yellow cupped flowers. Good for colonising nooks and crannies, say in a path or at the base of a wall. Likes a well-drained soil. It is drought-tolerant, so some will still be flowering when you return at the end of the summer holidays. Can become a nuisance if left to self-seed too freely.

Cornflower (Centaurea cyanus) Typically dark-blue, button-sized flowers on upright, greeny-grey stems. Will attract butterflies and bees.

Cosmos bipinnatus Single, elegant flower on top of delicate, feathery foliage. It can grow up to 1.5m, so grow in a clump so that plants support each other. Deadhead regularly to keep it flowering.

English marigold (Calendula officinalis) Also known as the pot marigold, this comes in yellow or orange and looks lovely self-seeding among the vegetables.

French marigold (Tagetes) Compact plant that will require more care than its English namesake and should definitely be started indoors. Often grown as a companion to greenhouse tomatoes, to deter whitefly. Try the Disco Series with its reddish-orange and yellow flowers with rich dark-brown markings.

Love-in-a-mist (Nigella) Saucer-shaped, typically sky-blue flowers above bushy foliage. Again, after establishing it in the garden, it can be left to self-seed where there is space.

Nasturtium (Tropaeolum majus) Looks good scrambling over a fence, hedge, path or shed roof rather than sat in a border. Bushy dwarf versions such as the Tom Thumb series are good for containers, and as a companion for crops that are susceptible to blackfly: not to deter them, but as an alternative host. Its edible, peppery-tasting leaves are best in very small quantities in a mixed salad.

Opium poppy (Papaver somniferum) Comes in a huge range of colours from white, through red to deep purple. The flowers vary tremendously from delicate single blooms to the great ruffs of the peony style. They can grow into large plants about 1m high and their flowers are short-lived, so best to leave them dotted around rather than let them take over.

Poached egg plant (Limnanthes douglasii) Has masses of yellow flowers with a white rim that are loved by bees and hoverflies. It self-seeds freely and is one to start off outside. Doesn't mind a bit of shade, either.

Sunflower (Helianthus annuus) This is unlikely to flower before the end of term, but is fun to grow. Keep it in a pot and the children can take it home to plant out during the summer term. Russian Giant is the real beast of legend, while for something different, try Velvet Queen, a smaller, red sunflower (yep, you heard right) with a dark brown centre. Remember, plants will need staking.

PROS

- A cheap and quick way to fill the garden full of flowers.
- Plenty of easy options for you.
- Many will self-seed freely after the first year.

CONS

- Self-seeding annuals can take over at the expense of other plants.
- In early spring, it can be difficult to distinguish between young, self-seeded annuals and weeds.

Spring

Don't forget ...

- Plant out autumn-sown sweet peas at the end of March/early April.
- Weeds will be starting to appear now. Get rid of them before they take over.
- March and early April are a good time to mulch the ground before it gets too dry and weeds get established.

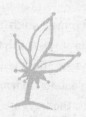

WEEK SIX

Leaf for spring

During the first year of the gardening club, the school kitchen stopped committing itself to a specific vegetable on its daily menu, and 'seasonal vegetables or salad' would most often appear instead. This not only made sense from a financial point of view – buying in what is seasonal and in plentiful supply – but it also meant gardening club salad got a warmer reception in the kitchen than it had previously.

With the exception of rocket, which is so quick to grow and does not seem attractive to our slugs, at this time of year we sowed our salad leaf in seed trays or modules, away from pests, then transplanted it when big enough to fend for itself. Unless specified otherwise on the packet, the trays are best kept indoors so your salad gets a good head start.

Sow salad little and often to ensure a constant supply and reduce gluts. It can be harvested when immature as baby leaves, so you can grow several varieties to create a mixed-leaf salad. Or it can be planted out after the Easter holidays and left to mature.

Which varieties to grow?

Lettuce: We didn't bother with the butterhead types as their soft leaves wilt soon after picking. Instead we grew 'Webb's Wonderful', lollo rosso, oak leaf and cos Little Gem. The iceberg-style lettuce Saladin was also very successful.

Lamb's lettuce (also known as mache or corn salad): Can be sown from March outdoors, it is so tough. Under cover, however, it will crop even earlier.

Rocket: This is a doddle to grow and best cultivated at the beginning or the end of the season, before the flea beetle is active. This nibbles rocket, leaving tiny but visible holes all over the leaf, as though it has been shot at with a miniature machine gun. Rocket grown in hot summer conditions also bolts easily. From the children's point of view, rocket's hot flavour makes it one of the least palatable salads. But it's expensive to buy, so is a good one for children to take home or sell at school. You can also sow 'wild' rocket, which is a short-lived perennial with narrower leaves and a sharper taste that will really impress any foodies among the parents. The irony is that once established, it is difficult to get rid of, with a tap root that goes deep into the earth. It will grow in shade, and can be cropped into winter, but keep it away from other plants and don't let it go to seed.

Mizuna: A Japanese green with serrated leaves that grows as easily as salad rocket, but has a milder flavour. A possible one for the kitchen.

PROS

- Always nice to have fresh salad at any time of year.

CONS

- Slower to get going at this time of year than later in the season.

Don't forget ...

🍂 You could sneak in a quick row of mangetout peas now, as well as after the holiday.

How will you look after the seed trays and pots over the Easter holidays? Here are some ideas:

1) If the forecast is for poor weather, you can get away with sitting the seed trays and pots in shallow trays with water in them. With a polytunnel or greenhouse, leave one door half-open unless frost is forecast. If they are being kept in a classroom, move away from direct sunlight on the windowledge, but put them somewhere where it is light. It would be best, though, if you could pop in half way through the break to check up on everything.

2) Is there a problem with access to the school over the holidays? If so, can you take the trays home with you?

3) If hot weather is expected and you have seed trays in the polytunnel, can you organise a watering rota among the children? A water every other day should do. Ask for volunteers, then talk to their parents, explaining that they only need honour their commitment if it is really hot. You should be able to muddle through.

Cut-and-come-again salad

Cut-and-come-again is the repeat harvesting of immature seedlings for salad, which then grow back again. Apart from loads of cheap, organic salad leaves to eat, cut-and-come again salad has added benefits in the context of a school because you get more than one harvest from the same crop – and harvesting, as any child will tell you, is one of the best things about growing.

There are many salad leaves that respond to this, but you can also use the young leaves of crops that would normally be cooked, such as Swiss chard and kale (see next page for a full list).

In the spring term, sow cut-and-come-again salad inside, in trays or in the ground in the polytunnel or greenhouse. Cut-and-come-again leaves do not take up much room, are happy in a pot or seed tray, and are remarkably productive where there is limited space. Larger seeds, such as lettuce, should be about 1cm deep; smaller seeds need just a smattering of soil above them. Make an indentation in the compost, water first, then sow seeds about 1cm apart.

One sowing of cut-and-come-again salad should be good for at least three harvests, but to ensure a continuous supply through the summer term, make another sowing in the first weeks, and another one towards the end of May – more if you have room or demand for your crop – there's nothing wrong with the children taking a bag of fresh leaves home with them each week. After the Easter holidays, the soil should be warm enough to have a go at sowing cut-and-come-again straight into the ground. Sow your salad-to-be into drills about 10cm wide. The site needs to be

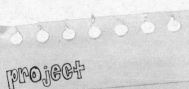

project

Create stripes or other patterns of cut-and-come-again crops by sowing alternating rows of leaves of different colours and shapes. Colourful leaves include red mustard, red orach and oak leaf lettuce. Green leaves? Well, you're spoilt for choice.

weed-free – you wouldn't want grass and baby thistles in your lunch, would you?

It is vital that your leaf is kept regularly watered over the summer to stop the plants bolting and, in the case of some of the stronger-tasting leaves such as red mustard and rocket, preventing them from becoming too fiery.

Your baby leaves are ready for cutting when about 6–10cm high. Cut them with scissors, always above the two leaves closest to the ground, leaving about 2cm of the plant behind. Now water and prepare for your next crop ... and the next ... and maybe even one or two more.

When to sow

Cut-and-come-again salad can be sown from March to September, outdoors weather permitting, or indoors at either end of the season.

Some lettuce and leaf varieties are tough enough to overwinter but would fare better in a cold greenhouse or polytunnel, or under a cloche outside.

Baby leaves to sow in cooler weather:

Salad rocket, mizuna, texsel greens, Russian kale, perpetual spinach (spring and early summer only), curly endive, choy sum, corn salad, oak leaf lettuce, red mustard, winter purslane, spinach (tricky to develop to a full-size crop but worth sowing as cut-and-come-again in cool weather).

Baby leaves to sow in warmer weather:

Red orach, bull's blood beet, chard, salad bowl and cutting lettuce varieties, summer purslane (requires warm weather).

PROS

- A cheap, easy and high-value crop: eat in school as a sophisticated garnish with the meal (no more watery iceberg and raw onion); use it to swell gardening club coffers and sell at the school gates; take it home to impress the family.
- Several harvests from the same crop in a single term.

CONS

- So much choice: where will you plant it all?

Spring term is also for ...

Sowing leeks

Leeks take a long time to reach maturity, during which period there is nothing else you can do with the ground they are in and, let's face it, they are not high on the list of children's vegetable must-haves. However, they are very easy to cultivate and will provide a gardening club with something to crop in the winter months: if you have enough room to grow them, ask the children what they think; let them vote on it. The leeks can always be secretly incorporated into a stew or hotpot at school lunchtime, and you can point out to the students that they make wonderful flowers if you are not growing them for food: large purple globes on top of thick 1m stems.

Which varieties to grow?

Leeks can be started off indoors or outdoors, depending on the particular cultivar and when you intend to harvest it. Starting them off indoors in March and then transplanting into the ground should eliminate competition from weeds and disruption by pests, resulting in strong plants able to survive the summer holiday. It should also give them the warmth they require to germinate well (10–15°C). Suitable varieties include Musselburgh, Toledo and Porsito.

Plant leeks 2cm deep in modules, about three per module. They will be ready to plant out in about 12 weeks, when pencil-thick, according to tradition, or 20cm tall.

PROS

* **Easy to grow and mostly pest-free.**
* **Something to harvest in the dead of winter.**

CONS

* **A very long growing season, so there will be nothing else you can do with the space in the meantime.**
* **For decent-sized leeks, they will have to be left in the ground over the summer holidays.**

Sowing carrots

Somehow a vegetable garden does not seem complete without carrots, and yet they are not the easiest of vegetables to grow. We had a dilemma in our gardening club: the children were keen to grow carrots, probably one of the most familiar vegetables to them, yet I was not sure of putting them in our heavy clay ground, carrots preferring light, well-drained soil, so their tap roots can easily work their way downwards. Why risk disappointment, when there were so many other things we could raise successfully?

The decision was made for us when a nursery that aims to promote growing in schools gave us some baby plants that included carrots. Rocket Gardens (www.rocketgardens.co.uk) specialises in organic plug plants by post, and supplies surplus material free to primary schools around the country. Naturally enough, we had signed up to this.

Carrots have another enemy besides heavy soil – the carrot root fly, whose grubs burrow into the vegetable root underground.

However, you can to some extent prepare for this by putting up a physical barrier around your crops to prevent the low-flying pest getting to them (*see below*), or growing carrots in containers or beds at least 60cm off the ground. Planting onions either side is supposed to help, too, because the scent of the latter masks that of the carrots so the flies can't smell the carrots.

project
A simple barrier against carrot root fly

You'll need six pieces of wood about 80cm long and 4cm wide, but you can probably get away with four. Ask the children to bring in any scraps they can find at home; even sturdy sticks will do. Now drive these into the ground so that they form a frame that encloses your row(s) of carrots. Each post should stand firm with at least 60cm protruding from the ground. Ideally, you would now wrap a piece of horticultural fleece around the whole thing, and pin it at the top and bottom using drawing pins borrowed from the classroom. However, clear polythene will do, so see what you and the children can come up with at home.

Which varieties to grow?

One way to avoid problems with heavy soil is to sow short, round carrots that will not need to delve so deep into the ground. The children should like the novelty of these, too. Handily, such cultivars lend themselves to being planted early under cover (from mid-March), which should be ready for cropping in June. Carrots don't like to be transplanted, so it is best they are sown thinly in modules (no more than three seeds per module), then planted outside when the foliage is about 2.5cm high. If necessary, thin before planting out so that seedlings are around 2.5cm apart. Carefully snip off the top of the carrot rather than uprooting it and bury the thinning in the compost heap. It sounds paranoid, but the scent of crushed thinnings can attract the carrot fly and you really want to do your utmost to keep it away. Suitable round varieties include Parabell, Parmex and Early French Frame.

One more thing: carrots like a fertile soil, but don't fertilise it just before planting – this encourages the roots to fork. We found this out the hard way having manured our soil before planting our carrots out.

PROS
- A favourite vegetable for children to grow.
- Quick maturing.
- Easy in light, well-drained soil.

CONS
- Does not grow well in heavy soil.
- Carrot root fly can ruin a crop.

project
A willow tunnel

One of the plans for the poorly drained ground in our garden is to build on it a tunnel of living willow (Salix species), with perhaps a willow igloo at one end of it. This, it is hoped, will alleviate the marshy conditions that make it a no-go zone after heavy rain. The willow should serve two purposes. Firstly, because it is a thirsty plant, it will be a cheap way of draining what is terribly boggy ground. Secondly, it will be a feature for the school children to enjoy – assuming conditions are dry enough.

Willow weaving is a traditional industry in the West Country, which includes one of the UK's centres of willow production, the Somerset Levels. This flat, mysterious landscape of sluices, waterways and ditches was once regularly flooded from the Bristol Channel in the north. Willow growing, and crafts in this area, date back to the Iron Age, and pollarded willow trees still hold the banks of the ditches in place.

Willow is a tough plant, but if you live in an exceptionally dry spot, a willow structure is perhaps not for you. But for the rest of us, willow structures are easy to create and satisfying in that they don't take too long to make. Of course, there are elaborate creations that involve much skill in their making, but the point of something like this in a school is that its construction involves the children, too.

How to make a willow tunnel

You will need:

Willow whips

For uprights and diagonals, available from November to April, either direct from suppliers in willow growing areas such as the Somerset Levels, or by mail order (see below).

Thin rods of the flexible back maul (*Salix triandra*)

For weaving horizontally

Spade

Compost

Weed-suppressant matting

Bark mulch

Willow is sold in imperial lengths and metric weights, hence the mish-mash of the following measurements. The quantity of willow you need will depend upon how long you want to the tunnel to be. The uprights should be spaced about 15cm apart, or about seven per metre, so for a 3m tunnel, 42 uprights should suffice. The length of the willow uprights will depend on how high you want the tunnel to be: 10ft stems will make a tunnel to walk through; shorter stems will do for crawling space.

You will also need the same amount again of shorter whips (8ft long if you have 10ft uprights) to weave in diagonally between the uprights, and about 1kg of thin rods known as triandra. The latter are woven horizontally along the tunnel, about halfway up the sides, again helping to strengthen the structure.

Suitable whips for living willow comes in different colours, from olive green (*Salix triandra*) to red, so why stick to one variety?

Mark out where the sides of the arch are to be and dig two narrow parallel trenches 15–20cm deep. Allow at least 1m between the trenches – enough to take a wheelbarrow if it is going to be a walkway.

Now fill the trenches with compost and firm down gently.

Push two willow uprights into the compost in opposite trenches, and tie them with twine at the top to make an arch. Repeat at 15cm intervals, keeping two of these long pieces aside at the end.

Now push the diagonal whips into the compost at the base of each upright, and weave them through the uprights. Continue weaving in 8ft diagonals to make a lattice effect. Cut and tie in when they join the top.

Tie the remaining two upright whips along the apex of the arch.

Weave in a thick band of the triandra about halfway up either side of the arch. This will help to strengthen the structure while the uprights grow their roots.

Give the base of the willow a good soak.

Finally, cut out strips of the matting wide enough to cover the compost. Line it up alongside the base of the willow and cut slits in it to take the willow stems. Now slide the matting across the compost and cover with the mulch.

In its first season, water the willow during hot or prolonged dry spells.

Living willow suppliers include PH Coate & Sons (01823 490249; www.livingwillow.net). Your supplier should give advice on quantities of willow needed for the structure you are planning. Some even provide living willow kits for a range of structures.

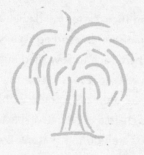

summer term

Children return from their Easter holiday in April, although the exact date will vary radically, depending on when Easter itself falls. At this time, it will be a race to sow seed and plant out flowers and veg so that you will see results before the end of term. Some crops, such as lettuce, are easy to raise within this time frame. Others, such as Swiss chard and perpetual spinach, are fine cropped and eaten when they are not fully mature. But with other crops, such as courgettes and French beans, you are cutting it fine and in some ways reliant on the weather.

You will be kept busy, also, with other jobs besides planting. Your plants will not be the only things to thrive with the onset of warmer weather and more light: weeds and pests will be on the move and will need to be kept at bay.

In other words, you might find the ten main activities outlined over the following pages to be too ambitious. If that is the case, you can always save some of them for next year. Ask the children what they would like to do each week. And don't forget to keep a journal. It will help you to build on your experiences this term and make gardening club more successful in the future.

WEEK ONE

Sow peas (or perhaps not)

By rights, peas should be in any child's vegetable plot. They are a core part of our diet – nothing weird or exotic about them – and many children love them. And it's likely they will really notice the difference between the sweet, fresh version straight from the pod and those from the freezer.

But the reality is that peas are difficult to grow. Though they are one of the vegetables that tolerate sowing early in the year, they suffer a high casualty rate, and so can be a disappointment. They are intolerant of hot weather, will not forgive you if you do not support them the moment they start growing, and are prone to many diseases. They are one of those plants that demand exactness from you: the right variety is needed for the correct sowing date; no compromising here, no room for manoeuvre.

That's the traditional garden pea. Mangetout-type peas, on the other hand, are a totally different story, being much easier to grow. They germinate quickly and, with the right variety, you can sow them outdoors from late March. A repeat sowing either side of the Easter holiday should be cropping from June onwards.

Sow the seeds in a zigzag pattern in a trench 15cm wide and 6cm deep, with 5cm between seeds, and water well while they are growing. If sowing more than one row, these should be 75cm apart.

As soon as the first tendrils appear on the plant, they will need support. At school, I got the children to tie twine between two bamboo canes at either end of the row, but this was not strong enough. Next time it will be wire, or mesh between sturdy posts. See if there is any of the ubiquitous green plastic fencing lying around at school, or ask the children whether they have something similar at home. As long as it is firmly held in place, it will do just fine.

Mangetout taste fabulous raw or cooked (before eating, remember to peel off the thin stringy layer on the inner semi-circle of the pod). They are ready to crop when about 5cm long and the seed peas inside are just beginning to show; later in the season, the seeds will get larger, when they can be shelled like normal peas. That's if they make it that far: the mangetout we grew didn't make it beyond our vegetable beds, the children preferring to pick and eat them straightaway. Next year, however, we intend to grow more – this is definitely one crop that should be served up in the kitchen.

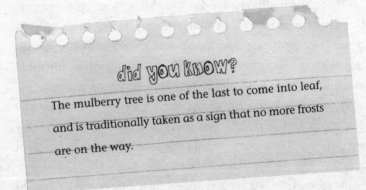

did you know?

The mulberry tree is one of the last to come into leaf, and is traditionally taken as a sign that no more frosts are on the way.

Which varieties to grow?

We had such success with Delikata that we're sticking with it.
Oregon Sugarpod comes highly recommended, too.

PROS

- Quick and easy, providing young plants can escape slugs
  and snails.
- Little in the way of pests and disease to worry about.

CONS

- If you're planning this for the kitchen, you'll have to stop
  the children gobbling up the crop as they pick it.
- Birds can be a problem with young plants, but the
  support should act as a deterrent.

Don't forget ...

🌱 Plant out beetroot: the soil should be warm enough now.

🌱 Check over the sweet peas and tie them into their supports.

🌱 Have tomatoes sown in trays been pricked out to small pots?

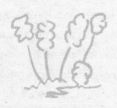

WEEK TWO

Sow leaf beet

Here, we are talking about Swiss chard and perpetual spinach, both members of the beetroot family that are grown for their leaves. Joy Larkcom, vegetable guru and someone to whom any grower should defer, has the following to say about Swiss chard: it's an 'ideal vegetable for beginners and absentee gardeners, as it withstands neglect and maltreatment well'. In other words, then, it gets my vote.

Swiss chard tastes fabulous, too. If you have been disappointed in this department, it is probably because it has been cooked whole. The trick is to separate stem and leaf, and give the former, the rib, a few more minutes in the pot.

Swiss chard has easy-to-handle, knobbly seeds the size of peppercorns, and can be sown outdoors from April onwards. It is slow to germinate, so be patient. Sow in rows about 35cm apart, thinning seedlings to 30cm between plants. If it is not fully mature by the end of term, it does not matter: young chard can be used as a cut-and-come-again salad. If left to mature, it is harvested by cutting off individual leaves from the main plant. Chard is so tough it will probably stay the distance of the summer holidays, waiting for you on your return in September and giving the gardening club interesting fresh greens to show off. You should be cropping Swiss chard well into winter and while it is not an obvious one to cook or disguise for school lunches, it is a good thing to sell at the school gates.

Both Swiss chard and perpetual spinach are members of the beetroot family and the latter's leaf is similarly robust. True spinach is difficult to grow in warmer months, being prone to bolting and a favourite of slugs and snails. Perpetual spinach, on the other hand, is a doddle, which makes it a good candidate for a school vegetable garden.

Perpetual spinach has coarser leaves than true spinach and if left to mature will have stems that might need a little more cooking

Summer

Windowsill planting

Here are some tips for raising seeds on a windowsill

1) Young seedlings can be scorched by full-on sun, so try to grow plants on a north-facing windowsill or, on a south-facing sill, put up some shading. This can simply be a sheet of thin white paper stuck to the glass.

2) Seedlings should be as close to the glass as possible. If too far away, they will not get enough light and become drawn and leggy as they grow towards the light.

3) As seedlings grow, you can rotate them once a day so that both sides get the best light.

4) Alternatively, you can keep the pots in a cardboard box with the side facing the window cut away and the back covered in kitchen foil to reflect the light.

5) If the central heating is still being used in the school, keep the plants away from the radiator.

than the main leaf. Like chard, it has knobbly seeds that are easy to handle, and its vigour and agreeable nature means you should try to go for a repeat sowing if a spare patch of ground comes available. Again like its cousin, you can use it for cut-and-come-again leaves when small, or leave it to mature.

In April, sow in drills outdoors, 10cm apart, thinning out if you require any plants to grow to full maturity. At the end of term, leave any plants where they are and some, if not all, should make it through to next term. If left alone, perpetual spinach will be cropping the following year, although less vigorously; pull it up when you need the space.

Which varieties to grow?

Many varieties of chard are pretty – Ruby chard and Bright Lights for example – so growing them should appeal to the children, if they are not totally convinced about the taste. They are a good choice for a potager, where vegetables are planted for their ornamental effect, or grown in a flowerbed. It is the green varieties, however, that are the best to eat. Try White Silver.

Perpetual spinach, meanwhile, is often sold as just that, or sometimes simply leaf beet.

PROS

* Some Swiss chard is beautiful in a garden, as well as on the plate.
* Swiss chard and perpetual spinach are both tolerant of light shade.
* Perpetual spinach is much easier to cultivate than true spinach.
* Both are drought tolerant, so could get through a summer holiday to provide fresh greens in the autumn.

CONS

* Touch and go as to whether they'll be fully mature by the end of term.
* Chard is prone to bolting if started off too early; leave sowing until April.
* Spinach is the probably the main vegetable children will not eat – come back, Popeye!

Don't forget ...

* Don't leave it too late to plant out carrots: the roots hate being disturbed.
* Mid-April is a good time to sow courgette and pumpkin seeds indoors.

WEEK THREE

French beans

Call me prejudiced, but I can't understand why runner beans are so popular. I always find them stringy. It might be bad luck on my part (Polestar and White Lady are reputed to be reliably unstringy), or it could be that runner beans are just more tricky to get right than their advocates insist. However, I think their popularity is also due to the fact that one plant will produce a massive crop and it feeds that very British appetite for quantity over quality.

Either way, why take the chance, especially when you have French beans waiting in the wings? The French bean helped to convert both my young daughters to the delights of green veg. I admit that one of them is on the verge of lapsing, but I comfort myself with the thought that had I tried to interest her in runner beans, we wouldn't even be where we are now. The chances of an unpalatable, stringy bean were just too high to risk her on runners: even if she had escaped a nasty experience with them, she would surely have picked up on my nervousness and become suspicious.

The children will enjoy growing French beans, which have pretty flowers in white, pink or red and lush foliage. When the climbers get into their stride in the warmer weather, it is real Jack and the Beanstalk stuff, the rampant tendrils racing skywards. 'You'll be lucky to get them that big,' said one of the lunchtime supervisers as the children and I put up a bean frame some 2.5m high. By the end of the summer she had to eat her words.

Which varieties to grow?

French beans come as either dwarf plants or climbers: the former crop slightly more quickly than the latter and take up less space (try Kenyan, or for interesting bean colour, the yellow Rocquencourt or Purple Tepee). Climbers, on the other hand, are more prolific (at gardening club, we swear by the variety Blue Lake, not blue-coloured beans alas, but masses of ordinary green ones). As flowers begin to form, spread the word among the children: the plants will need to be watered well to get good beans for cropping.

French beans are usually safe to plant straight into the ground as seeds in early May, when the soil has warmed up (to 10°C), but are susceptible to cold weather which could knock them back or even kill them. Slugs and snails love them, too. It is best, then, if you have an eye on a crop before the summer break, to sow them indoors in pots (mid-April) and plant them out when large enough to have a fighting chance against pests. Sow more than you think you will need, then any that get eaten by slugs can be replaced. A surplus can be given away.

Sow seeds in 10cm pots, 5cm deep. Plant out when 10cm tall, allowing at least 25cm between plants each way. It is important to support beans at all stages of their life; use small sticks when they are young. Dwarf plants in double rows will support each other to some extent, but the children could gather twiggy branches to lay alongside the plants and act as extra support: this will also help to deter birds.

Climbing plants need a structure, such as a wigwam, which should ideally be in place before they are planted out. Allow one plant per cane, which should be at least 1.8m out of the ground. In rural areas, you might be able to get hold of coppiced hazel sticks which make lovely frames for your beans. But despite their rustic appearance and timeless quality, they are likely to be much pricier than bamboo canes, which our garden centre sells for 35p for a 2m length.

French beans do best on light, well-drained soils that retain moisture well. Planting in ground prepared with compost the previous autumn will help them while they are growing.

These beans are ready to harvest when they can be snapped in half; regular picking will ensure a heavy crop.

A quick Latin lesson

Why do plant names have to be in Latin? The answer is so that everyone can recognise the exact plant we are talking about, whether they be in Kew or Kuala Lumpar. Take the poppy. Its Latin name is *Papaver*, which describes the genus, but this does not tell us much. There are many different poppies in the world, some better suited than others to specific climate and habitat. However, *Papaver orientale* narrows down the particular poppy we are talking about to a poppy species, in this case the oriental poppy. There are still plenty of oriental poppies out there, so how do we distinguish one from another? This is the bit that comes after the Latin name and is in single quotation marks; it is what is known as the cultivar and denotes a specific plant that has been bred by a gardener.

PROS

- **Colourful crop that holds interest in every stage of development.**
- **Children love to eat them.**

CONS

- **If caught by a late cold snap, you might not be able to crop them before the end of term. Don't plant out until the weather is fine.**
- **The taller varieties need support structures – if supports are hard to source, grow dwarf varieties.**
- **Adored by slugs and snails – take precautions.**

Don't forget ...

- Have you sown more cut-and-come-again salad in trays to transplant? If the weather is mild, you could now try some outdoors.
- If sunflowers have germinated, remember they will need supporting.
- Annuals grown indoors can be hardened off and planted out from early May. Avoid doing this if frost is forecast.
- Protect your strawberry plants from birds (*see protecting onions, page 243*).

WEEK FOUR

Plant bedding for summer containers

At school, there is a cluster of large pots next to the entrance that have become the gardening club's responsibility. By early summer term, any spring bulbs that have been planted in them will have died off or be hanging on for dear life. Time, then, for action.

Handily, by late April, the garden centres are full of young 'plug' plants that are ideal for a summer container. They will often be described as bedding plants, which means flowering or foliage ornamentals designed for a summer display, and are designed to belt out colourful blooms in the shortest possible time.

Compared to the price of a packet of seed, they are expensive – prices vary tremendously but I expect to pay around £3–£4 for a tray of 12 plugs – but they are just the quick fix a gardening club needs. Also, compared to the price of other plants you buy ready-grown, they can seem like a bargain: remember that these tiny plants will get much bigger, so work that into your calculations. In our case we are lucky: the head teacher is very happy to pay £10 or so for a bright display in front of her school; either that or she has to look at dying spring bulbs every morning on her way to work. You might soon have profits from selling some of your vegetables, so maybe you could shell out a bit of money now in anticipation of riches to come.

Alternatively, try contacting local garden centres and nurseries, explaining that you want spare bedding plants for containers, and could they spare any in exchange for a mention in the school newsletter? You will be surprised at how many will be more than happy to help.

Which varieties to grow?

The short answer here is choose whatever is on sale at the garden centre. If you want to go to the trouble, get a list so students can Google the plants, then decide for themselves. There are a growing number of mail order suppliers of plug plants, too (try Thompson & Morgan, http://plants.thompson-morgan.com) but check how long they will take to arrive: you can't wait around for those containers to be filled.

Ten bedding plants for summer

Ageratum Compact mound-forming plant with small flowers that form clusters. Usually comes in blue, so very tasteful as far as bedding goes.

Antirrhinum The good old snapdragon with its spires of lipped flowers will appeal to children, so planting them might have to come with a strict warning not to play with them. They look lovely in a swathe of one colour, but are often sold in mixed colours. If you really want the sweet-shop effect, look for the yellow and red 'Bicolour': just like the rhubarb and custard boiled sweets.

Begonia The begonias sold as bedding in the garden centre are a mere fraction of a huge genus that includes houseplants grown for their interesting foliage. But let's focus on those plugs at the garden centre: these will often turn into flouncy,

195

double-flowered blooms in hurt-your-eyes colours. You'll be lucky if you can find any sold in one colour, so prepare to throw good taste to the wind. The 'pendulous' varieties are good for dangling from a hanging basket.

Gazania Large, daisy-like flowers in oranges, yellow and reds and with a dark centre. They are happy in an exposed site and their drought tolerance is handy if you forget to water the containers.

Geranium Strictly speaking, a pelargonium. A popular plant to grow in single pots on the window ledge, but equally at home outdoors in a summer container. Clusters of flowers on upright stems, typically in shades of pink or red. If you keep them indoors over winter, then cut them back in February, you'll have plants again next year, though with woody stems. It is easy to take cuttings from pelargoniums, too.

Impatiens Better known as the busy Lizzie, this is sniggered at by many as a naff little bloom, preferred by ladies of a certain age. But not only are busy Lizzies cheap, they tolerate shade, too.

Pansy Pansies planted at this time of year, as opposed to autumn, will expand, but could get overwhelemed if too close to more boisterous neighbours such as petunias. Deadhead the moment you see flowers fading and these will go on and on.

Petunia Masses of mostly saucer-shaped blooms, this is a bedding favourite. The cascading types are often sold as 'surfina'. Pinks, reds and mauves are typical.

Salvia Salvia bedding comes from a huge extended family that includes sage and many popular perennials in the herbaceous border. Small spires of individual flowers above compact, bushy foliage. Often sold in a single colour – red is typical – so one to go for if the clashing tendency of many bedding plants is not your thing.

Zinnias These can get really gaudy, but are outrageous and fun. There are less in-your-face combinations and more modest, daisy-style flowers, too, but they're not for the faint-hearted.

Most plants – flower, vegetable or even tree – can go into a container, as long as it is big enough. One important thing to remember is that though some plants might not have significant roots, meaning they can fit into relatively small pots, if they get too big they will topple over – sunflowers are a good example.

Containers should be kept watered, too and the bigger they are the longer they will take to dry up. Children love watering, but will they remember to check all the pots, all the time? Your pots will need to be fed, also, to ensure these concentrated islands of colour to perform their best throughout the term.

PROS

- Plug plants are a quick fix for summer containers.
- Bedding plants are tricky to raise from seed – here the hard work is done for you.

CONS

- Much more expensive than raising seed yourself.
- You are stuck with an often limited range at the garden centre or from mail order – and these are often in gaudy colours.

project

The strange container show

Ask students to make a plant container out of any object, plant it up and bring it into school. The results will then be displayed around the school for the rest of term. Remind children that the container should have some drainage holes and preferably crocks or old stones in the bottom of it. When we did this at school, some of the entries included a hat, an old wellie and a child's wheelbarrow.

This is something to organise for the whole school, if you can get the teachers behind you. It can be open to every student, as it was with ours, but if you are in a large school it could become too unwieldy and you might want to limit it to one container per class, the children bringing in necessary materials to plant up.

Don't forget ...

- The annuals you planted last term should be growing nicely now. Most of these are ideal for a container, so could be an alternative to ready-made bedding. Cornflowers, for example, look beautiful planted in a mass, while nasturtiums are perfect for dangling from a hanging basket.

- Water the beetroot: a silly thing to point out, perhaps, given the number of willing hands at your disposal, but this time of year the ground will be drying out if not watered and dry ground could mean a harvest of woody beets.

WEEK FIVE

May is for lettuce

As the weather of the summer term gets warmer and the days get longer, some salad leaf will not be performing at their best. The oriental greens, for example, germinate better from August sowings when days are shorter, and grow well in the cool of early autumn. Spinach has a tendency to bolt in warm weather – rocket, too.

But this is lettuce time, when you can practically watch these plants growing on a daily basis. It is nice, then, to leave some lettuce to grow to full maturity, as well as having your cut-and-come-agains – the hearting types to swell into firm centres surrounded by a ruff of looser leaves, like a child's picture of the sun; the looseleaf varieties to gently unfurl like the petals of a giant flower. These make perfect gifts from children to their parents.

Lettuce and salad leaves are wonderfully versatile, and their quick maturing make them ideal for a school gardening club. As your lettuces grow, an alternative way of cropping them is to pick off mature leaves from the outside as you need them.

Now, early in the summer term, lettuce sowings can go straight into the ground, as recommended on seed packets, but if started outdoors in trays, modules or pots that are raised off the floor, they will have more chance against pests.

In hot weather, lettuce germination can be erratic. You can get round this in several ways:

Sow in the afternoon so that soil is cooler during the critical germination stage a few hours later. However, this can be tricky if, like us, your gardening club meets at lunchtime. Our solution then was to plant varieties that were not so demanding. Plant crisphead cultivars that include the Cos types (Little Gem is a winner) and Iceberg types (these are not always the bland, watery heads you get at the supermarket). Other popular varieties include Webb's Wonderful, Reine Des Glaces, Triumph, Chartwell and Rubens.

Sow in seed trays and put in a cool place until germination has taken place. Transplant to their final position when the seedlings are about 5cm high – preferably when it is not too hot and out of the glare of the sun.

Sow your lettuce in partial shade where seedlings are not going to be exposed to the full force of the sun.

Lastly, water the ground before sowing, to cool it down.

PROS

- **You can never have enough salad.**

CONS

- **All that salad you are growing might put children off for life.**
- **Slugs and snails will still be a problem – don't get complacent.**

Don't forget ...

- If growing tomatoes outdoors, plant out at the end of May. If growing indoors, this can be done sooner. And don't forget to feed them regularly.
- Leeks raised indoors can go outside in their seed trays in May.

WEEK SIX

Sow basil: the herb for summer

There is a small crowd at gardening club who are obsessed with pesto. I know this because my daughter is the ringleader. If she had her way, she would eat it most of the time, with the occasional break for Shreddies, a boiled egg or fish fingers. When she was very young and refusing to eat most of her fruit and vegetables, it amused me that one of her favourite foods was largely made up of basil (that's when I wasn't worrying about her going down with scurvy). What would she do if she knew that pesto didn't come from a jar? That it was really made up of green leaves and grew in the same place as cabbage and sprouts?

Actually, when she did find out the truth about pesto a couple of years later, she took it rather well (her diet had diversified slightly and certain veg were being eaten without much drama). Likewise, her peers at gardening club were similarly cool about this revelation. All the more reason, then, for us to grow it.

Basil needs warmth, the warmer the better. Seed packets say that you can start it indoors, and when it is hot enough, transplant it outside. If you have a polytunnel, or any sunny inside space, I say, 'Don't bother.' Put it with the tomatoes in the polytunnel, raise it in pots, then take it home or sell it.

There are several types of this most delicious herb to tempt you when buying seeds, including Greek, purple-leaved, lemon-flavoured varieties and the extraordinary Thai basil. The latter, added just before you serve up, will make a dish of stir-fried noodles or hot coconut curry into something truly special. But at gardening club we stuck to the reliable and versatile sweet basil, *Ocimum basilicum* 'Genovese'. This needs a temperature of 15–20°C to germinate.

Basil has a long tap root and hates being moved so sow in modules or pots, three seedlings to an 8cm pot. Don't try to emulate the pot herbs you buy in the shops, where several seedlings are crammed into a small container: basil is prone to damping off, the fungal disease that kills seedlings when they are overcrowded and in an over-humid atmosphere, so sowing them cheek by jowl is only inviting trouble.

Water plants during the middle of the day, so that the compost is not too wet by nightfall. As your basil grows, pinch out the tops of young plants to encourage new leaf growth. Harvest from the top down, which will also promote new growth.

Basil can stay in the pots in which they were sown, or join more plants in larger containers. A healthy, bushy plant in a terracotta pot makes a nice fundraiser or end-of-term present for teacher or the family.

PROS

* **Perfect for growing in containers.**
* **Easy to grow in warm conditions.**
* **Makes lovely presents.**

CONS

* **Much better grown indoors.**
* **Seedlings are susceptible to damping off, a fungal disease**

Summer

project
Classic pesto Genovese

So no one believes that you can make pesto as good as that in the jar? Here's how to prove them wrong. You will need:

2 adult handfuls of basil leaves

2 cloves of garlic, peeled

10g pine kernels

50g Parmesan cheese, finely grated or better, 30g
  Parmesan and 20g Pecorino

60ml olive oil

Salt

Large mortar and pestle

With the mortar and pestle, crush together salt, garlic and a few of the basil leaves. Keep adding basil until it is nicely incorporated. Now add the pine kernels and keep working with the mortar and pestle until it forms a paste. Add cheese, then slowly pour in the oil, mixing all the time.

Top tip 1) It doesn't taste like the pesto from the supermarket? Add more salt: this is the trick with many of the recipes you find in a jar.

Top tip 2) Borrow a blender and do away with the mortar and pestle altogether.

caused by overcrowded seedlings kept in wet conditions. Sow seed thinly to help prevent it.

- **Greenfly and whitefly can be a problem. If it becomes a real problem, try biological controls (visit www.organiccatalog.com).**

Don't forget ...

Pumpkins will be ready to plant out from mid-May when all risk of frost has passed. Are yours ready? If so, the children can take them home at the end of the session. Are you going to keep some back to grow on at gardening club (*see page 218*)?

Tie sweet peas to their supporting stakes to help them keep climbing upwards.

Will you be having a grand veg and flower sale later in the term? At our school, there are fewer windows of opportunity for such things as the term goes on and everyone gets busier. Assess the state of the garden now, and make plans. Maybe a Friday, tagged on to something else like a sports day or in the case of our school, the regular fund-raising cake sale.

WEEK SEVEN

Make a simple herb garden

If growing basil has given you an appetite for raising more herbs – as well as homemade pesto – summer is a good time to get a herb garden going. Many of our favourite perennial herbs are widely available as young plants, and very cheap, too. There are some (chives come to mind) that are easy to grow from seed, but with the popular woody evergreens thyme, rosemary, bay and sage, give yourself a head start and buy a plant from the garden centre. They will put on growth over the rest of the season and you shouldn't have to worry about watering them during the holidays – they hail from hot countries around the Mediterranean, so a British summer will be a walk in the park. They also don't mind poor soil, as long as it is well drained.

There is also enough time for you to grow more annual and biennial herbs, which could become part of your herb garden. But before you do, make sure there is a point to this: are they destined for the kitchen, to take home or to sell after school one day? At gardening club, we made the mistake of growing too much parsley and couldn't even give the stuff away.

Strictly speaking, a herb is a plant grown for its medicinal or flavouring properties, so a glance through my encyclopedia on the subject reveals a huge range of plants that could technically call themselves herbs – from cowslips (insomnia remedy) and houseleeks (treating burns and insect bites), to honeysuckle flowers (for salads) and monkshood (er, poisonous, so be very careful).

Inspired by this range, and with the exception of plants such as monkshood, you could grow a huge range of plants and call it an apothecary's garden.

For most of the herbs that you will want to grow for the kitchen, the ideal spot is an open, sunny site. Rosemary and thyme are used to baking on southern European hillsides, not shivering in the English shade. The original home of these herbs is also a clue to the soil they prefer – well-drained and with no danger of their roots sitting in water. Many of these herbs, then, lend themselves well to containers. And if ever there was an argument for a raised bed, it is here. Fill up your new herb garden with plenty of horticultural grit for drainage, and watch those plants go.

What herbs to plant?

Many of our favourite herbs are evergreens, so you could create a formal evergreen garden using them, with perennials to fill in any gaps. Thymes are useful here, as they come in different greens and variegated (ie white and green) forms. One popular perennial herb that does not like a hot, open site is mint. This prefers moist soil and doesn't mind a bit of shade. If planting this out, keep it in a generous-sized pot and bury the whole thing, with the top of the pot proud of the ground: mint is invasive and this will help to contain it.

Easy evergreens for the herb garden:

Bay: not fully hardy, so keep away from exposed sites.

Rosemary: generally hardy and flowers in colours from dark blue, through pink to white. Some varieties such as *Rosmarinus officinalis* 'Benenden Blue' have more needle-like leaves than others, so care has to be taken with cooking. Lovely, light blue types include 'Miss Jessop's Upright', which can be used for hedging, and 'Sissinghurst Blue'. Rosemary can give a second flush of flowers in late summer, but cutting back after first flowering will ensure it keeps it shape.

Sage: culinary sage belongs to the large salvia family and is reputed to be good for the brain, senses and memory, as well as being popular stuffed into a roast bird. Common sage, *Salvia officinalis*, has blue flowers in summer; 'Purpurascens' has purple leaves but is less hardy. Cut back hard after flowering in summer to retain the bushiness of the shrub and stop it becoming woody. You can also prune it in spring, but then risk losing summer flowers. Sage plants eventually become very woody and will probably need replacing every four or five years.

Thyme: an ancient herb used by the Romans and Greeks, and although associated with Mediterranean cultures, it is found as far north as Greenland, too. There are many species with their characteristic tiny leaves and flowers in pinks, white and red. With such a choice, it is best to see what the garden centre is selling and make your selection there. Some thymes have a creeping habit and are good fillers in paving cracks or hanging in walls; others form attractive little mounds that can be shaped after they have flowered.

Summer

Easy perennials for the herb garden:

Chives and garlic chives: grass-like and with a mild oniony flavour. Like a grown-up member of the allium family, it has lovely pink/purple flowers if left alone, though at this point the stems won't be good to eat. A really easy plant to raise from seed, and if sown a few weeks into the summer term, will be ready to harvest before the holidays. After dying off for winter, it will be back again early the following spring.

Marjoram: one to buy from the garden centre, as the majority of marjorams are propagated from cuttings or division.

Fennel: its feathery leaves in bronze or green grow on stems up to 1.5m high. It is a lovely sight in any part of the garden, with its flowerheads surrounded by insects in the summer and its tall silhouette lasting well into winter. It will seed all around the garden if allowed, so be sure you like it before you let it in. Again, one to grow from seed early in the summer term, or even better, save yourself the price of a seed packet and beg a root from another gardener. There will be plenty nearby digging up young fennel plants to throw on the compost heap.

This time next year, when your herb garden is established, you can harvest some of the herbs you have grown and dry them.

Don't forget ...

- Young leeks should be transplanted when they are the width of a pencil. Make holes 15–20cm deep and about 5cm across: at school we used the handles of a rake and hoe to do this. Now, gently ease the leek seedlings out of their compost, give one each to a child and get them to pop them into the holes. When planted, do not put soil back into the hole, but fill with water instead.

🍂 Your carrots should be ready to harvest in June. Strawberries too.

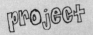

project

Make some dried herbs

This is ideal for the woody-stemmed herbs such as rosemary and thyme. Each child should cut off a few sprigs of the same herb, wash them in cold water, then leave them to dry on kitchen roll.

Once the herbs are dry, tie the stems together with a piece of string and put them upside down into a paper bag. Tie the top of the bag with the stems sticking out, then make some holes in the bag. This can now be taken home to hang in the airing cupboard and should be ready to use in a month.

Make your own bags of mixed herbs for selling at the school gate. A typical recipe will contain

3 tbsp dried marjoram

3 tbsp dried thyme

1 tsp dried basil

1 tsp dried rosemary

½ tsp dried sage

WEEK EIGHT

Grow microgreens to take home

They are barely a few centimetres high, and some look like grass cuttings, but so-called microgreens are to be found in some of the best restaurants in the world. Microgreens are tiny, highly nutritious vegetable seedlings that are valued by cooks because of their intense flavour. Raymond Blanc, Gordon Ramsay and Tom Aikens are some of the top-name chefs who swear by them.

Growing them is not rocket science, despite their technical sounding name. Microgreens (also known as microherbs and living greens) can be sown directly on to compost in a seed tray or pot, but it is better to use vermiculite from the garden centre. The container they grow in needs to be placed in a larger tray of water. Sow a generous amount of seed on to the vermiculite and add water to the tray until the vermiculite's surface is wet. Never water the seeds themselves: always water via the tray and keep the tray topped up with water.

Microgreens can be grown all year round on a sunny windowsill, so they are a good way to get a fix of fresh vegetables in the depths of winter (try them in gardening club next term, but expect them to take longer). In summer, they grow really quickly (cropping within seven to ten days), so you could wait for the seeds to germinate before sending them home with the children. Harvest with a pair of scissors.

Which varieties to grow?

Many vegetables make good microgreens, although reservations have been expressed about the suitability of parsnips. Snow peas, broccoli, radish, Swiss chard and beetroot are among the many veg you can grow in this way.

Don't forget ...

- Deadhead annual flowers that are fading to encourage them to produce more blooms.
- How are your potatoes looking? They will be ready to harvest when the flowers begin to die back.

Summer

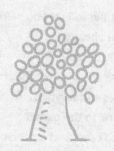

WEEK NINE

Make a hiding place for hoverflies and friends

Towards the end of the summer term, unless you have watering rotas set up for the long holiday or an irrigation system in place, there is little point in sowing things in the hope that they'll be alive when you come back for the autumn term. So what else to do?

Autumn is the traditional time for gardeners to make provision for wildlife in their patch, creating places for hiding and hibernation during the winter that is on its way. But it is actually a good thing to create some of those creature comforts now, because some of the wildlife in question will use it over the summer. Leave it until autumn and some of the insects you want to attract might have gone into hibernation already.

One simple thing that children can build, without the supervisory nightmare of hammers and sharp tools, is a 'hotel' for solitary bees, hoverflies and ladybirds. All are beneficial insects that you want to encourage in the garden.

Take some bamboo canes and cut them into lengths of between 20cm and 30cm (a 1m length of bamboo should set you back around 20p, so this should not be expensive). You should aim to end up with about 20 pieces for each hotel you intend to create. The canes you use should not be too small or narrow, either: you want to encourage insects inside them.

Now, tie the canes together using gardening twine or wire and secure, off the ground, in a sheltered spot (preferably near an aphid infestation). Ladybirds will take advantage of its shelter now, and possibly use it for hibernation in the winter, as will hoverflies. The hollowed-out canes also make an ideal place for solitary bees to lay their eggs.

An alternative – albeit an expensive one – is to buy a specially made wildlife hotel. The advantage here is that some of them come with viewing windows so that students can see what is going on inside. Check out www.greengardener.co.uk

Don't forget ...

- Get everything in place for next week's sale.
- Have the Christmas potatoes you ordered arrived? Dig them into the ground now for harvesting late next term.

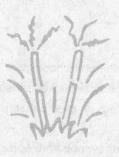

213

WEEK TEN

A harvest for the summer sale

After all the effort the children and you have put in over the season, gardening club should go out with a bang. Make sure you have set a date for a sale of remaining flowers and crops, preferably on the same day that gardening club meets, so that they are fresh from the soil. It will be tricky to time everything to be ready at once, and many vegetables might have been used up by the kitchen or taken home after school. But even a sale of half a dozen lettuce and some spuds is something to be proud of. The event can be as grand or as modest as you think fit and resources allow: perhaps the children could paint a banner on a giant piece of cardboard, announcing your stall of organically grown veg. And make signs identifying each of the veg.

> **You will need:**
> A table (borrow this from school)
> Old boxes from the supermarket to house your veg
> Bags (old carrier bags or, even better, paper ones)
> Price list
> Scales (can you borrow one from home or the kitchen?)
> A float and till (we used an old biscuit tin)
> Willing helpers

The children can bring in most things you will need – you just have to fix a time, a table, a float and permission for the gardening club to leave classes if needed for harvesting or staffing the shop. Try to set up somewhere in the shade, or even in the school building, so that your produce stays in the best condition possible.

Don't forget ...

- Just before the end of term, earth up leeks (gently push the soil up around the stems so you end up with more of the tasty white stalk) and give them a good soaking of water.
- Soak and mulch any pumpkins and leaf beet you are leaving behind for the summer.
- Cultivate open bits of ground by sowing green manure to keep down weeds.

Summer is also for ...

Courgettes

If they germinate well, if the weather is good to you, and if you plant them mid to late April indoors, you should be cropping courgettes before the end of term. That's a lot of ifs. However, many courgettes have a bushy habit and are reasonably compact, so you could hedge your bets and grow them to maturity in containers around 30–40cm in diameter, keeping them indoors for longer and only moving them outside for summer proper. Or you could experiment by growing some in pots and some in the ground, then comparing the results.

Once they are mature, courgettes are prolific croppers and one plant can produce 15–20 courgettes. In a container, this yield

Summer

might be reduced, but you will not need many plants for a decent-sized harvest.

The seeds must be sown in warm soil (13–15°C), so definitely start them off indoors, mid-April onwards. Plant seeds individually in small pots. Some gardeners say that the seeds must be planted on their sides for better germination, as opposed to being laid down flat, but we had a good hit rate with our courgette seedlings and I can guarantee not all of them went in this way.

When two leaves have formed and a third is starting to develop, your plants are ready to go outside. The timing of this is crucial, however. If cold weather is anticipated, you should keep the plants indoors, potting on if need be, or put them outside under cloches until decent late spring/summer weather really kicks in. If planting outside, dig a good-sized hole for your seedling and fill it with organic matter before planting, leaving about 30cm between plants. Courgettes are hungry plants – that is why they are often grown on top of the compost heap – and will reward you for giving them the extra boost.

Which varieties to grow?

The yellow Burpee's Golden, Venus and Zucchini are suitable for the container treatment, or growing on outdoors. Defender is recommended for early cropping. Courgettes come in fun shapes and sizes, too: Tromboncino is trombone-shaped, while De Nice a Fruit Rond is round.

Water well when fruits form and if growing in a container, feed once a fortnight (*see comfrey tea, page 37*). For flavour, courgettes are best harvested young, when firm to the touch and with their flowers still on them. Cut them using secateurs to avoid damaging the plant. Regular cropping is essential to encourage more fruit. For larger courgettes, you can wait until the flower begins to fade and can easily be knocked off. Leave them any longer to turn into marrows and they not only lose flavour, but cropping slows down too.

Summer

PROS

* Prolific plants – one will produce up to 25 courgettes.
* Will crop in summer term if grown indoors.
* Fun for children: makes an attractive plant in a container, with trumpet-shaped yellow flowers and attractive fruit.

CONS

* Snails and slugs love the young plants.
* Red spider mite could be a problem if grown on indoors.
* If grown outdoors, you risk having no fruit by the summer holidays.

Pumpkins (and winter squash)

If there is one vegetable that really captures a child's imagination, it has to be the pumpkin – though the reasons for this have more to do with Halloween than gardening. Still, you should not let this get you down. True, Halloween has become something of a commercial racket these days, with trick-or-treating children learning the principles of extortion from an early age, but a hollowed-out pumpkin, on the other hand, is a reminder of more innocent times.

We started our pumpkins and courgettes at the same time, and when the children were given the choice of what seeds we were going to sow, there was a huge rush for the former. No surprises there.

The problem for a gardening club, however, is that pumpkins (and winter squash) are slow burners, taking the whole summer to bulk up and ripen before harvest time in September and October. During this time they will need plenty of water, so even if a wet summer is predicted, it is a gamble leaving them for the holidays. Many of them take up loads of room, too, so unless you have a variety that you can train up a wall or over a pergola, they are not suited to a small garden.

Of course, as a gardening club, you could decide not to have pumpkins at all, but I think this would be a shame for the children, given their popularity and the almost cartoon-ish way they put on growth. One of the main points about pumpkins is that they are fun. The solution, I think, is to start them off in school and risk leaving two or three plants in heavily mulched ground over the summer holidays (perhaps someone among staff, parents and pupils could be persuaded to pop into school and water them, or you could set up a rota among the children). As for the rest of your seedlings – any child who wants one could take one home and report back on their success the following term.

Which varieties to grow?

Look online and in seed catalogues, and you'll see there are dozens of varieties to grow. I have read of one seasoned grower in Brighton whose ambition is to raise 100 different types of pumpkin and squash.

If you were opting for size above anything else, then you could go for Atlantic Giant, but the really huge pumpkins tend to lack flavour, some to the extent that they are inedible. A compromise candidate – and one that is good for carving and eating – is Small Sugar. Other flavoursome squash are Sunburst, a patty-pan variety shaped like a flying saucer, blue-skinned Crown Prince and Festival. A less vigorous butternut variety that is bushy rather than trailing is Pilgrim Butternut.

Like courgettes, pumpkins should be started off in mid-April indoors, and only put outside when all risk of frost has passed. They do not want their growth checked by cold weather.

Typically, they need about 2m diameter growing space, and should be planted out in a sunny, sheltered spot into fertile soil with good drainage. Trailing varieties such as Crown Prince and Festival can be trained up supports, but make sure the supports are strong and the fruit is supported when it forms. They can also be coiled round in a spiral on the ground to save space. Pumpkins are also very successful if grown on old compost heaps.

If you are trying to get the largest pumpkin possible, remove the growing tip once one fruit has formed – the plant can now put all its energies into producing a whopper. Otherwise, with cultivars with large fruit, stop the plant after three pumpkins have

Summer

formed by pinching out the growing tip.

Fruits should start to ripen in August, when you can cut away leaves that are shading them.

Harvesting pumpkins is an inexact science. With most winter squash, it is best to leave them on the plant to ripen for as long as possible, so keep your fingers crossed for a sunny September. Once you harvest them, and this should be before cold, wet autumn gets into its stride, leave your squash to 'cure' in a sunny sheltered spot, bringing it indoors if it rains. This will help the skin to harden, which you need if the squash is to store.

PROS

- **An absolute favourite with children.**
- **A good plant for the children to take home.**

CONS

- **Hungry feeders.**
- **Need plenty of water.**
- **Will not crop before the end of term.**

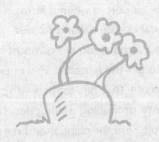

Summer

project

Dare you eat nettles?

Nettles might be infamous stingers, but they have many other uses. They can be mixed with water and turned into fertiliser; a nettlebed is a haven for insects; or you can make a nutritious soup from them.

You will need

Gloves for picking the nettles
Half a carrier bag of nettles (only the tops and leaves
  of young nettles, not the stalks)
1lb potatoes
2oz butter
1.5 pints vegetable stock
4 tablespoons of sour cream or crème fraiche
  or Greek yoghurt

Peel, chop and boil potatoes for 10 minutes. Drain and set aside.
  Wash and chop the nettles, then sweat in the butter in a heavy-bottomed saucepan
  Add potatoes and heated stock, bring to boil and simmer for 10 minutes. When the potatoes are cooked through, purée them, add salt, pepper and the sour cream and serve.

autumn term

Though the gardening year is drawing to a close in autumn, you can still be planting things for an early start in the spring. Broad beans are a good crop to sow and sweet peas are best got in at the end of October. There are other jobs in the garden such as sorting out the compost heap, organising bird feeders and clearing the beds of summer debris.

At this time of year, some sessions will inevitably be rained off. Despite the shelter of our polytunnel, when it's really filthy outside, the children always end up with mud on their clothing as they pop in and out of it. Our get-togethers are too short for the children to get changed into old clothes first, and as for wellies – I have as good as given up reminding them to bring them in. In other words, I don't expect gardening club to run regularly through the term, and the six activities outlined below will be spread over more than six weeks.

WEEK ONE

Bulbs – the big push

If there is one group of plants with which I most associate autumn, it has to be spring bulbs. In our local garden centre, pots of late-flowering perennials such as dahlias and penstemon are still in their prime when the daffodils, tulips and crocus bulbs have taken over the indoor section. It's a sobering reminder that, despite the fact that many gardens are still going strong and it's warm enough to have forgotten when you last wore a coat, it won't be that long before you are standing in November drizzle, cooing at the fireworks.

Bulbs are great things to plant with children because of their reliable results. There is something appealing about their size, too: perhaps it is more fun to put something so substantial in the ground. It is certainly easier to make a connection between a fine, swollen bulb of a hyacinth than a fiddly fleck of seed that you have to squint at to see properly.

Early September is just about OK to order from the mail order bulb companies in time to plant over the coming months. Aficionados, however, will have ordered their bulbs much earlier, probably around late July or early August, to guarantee they get exactly what they want and that it is good quality. I suspect the majority of gardeners are different; even if we are interested in buying mail order, we usually don't get round to it and end up taking whatever the garden centre has to offer.

The garden centre offerings will doubtless be extremely limited

Autumn

223

when set against the specialist suppliers, but there is one advantage. Here you can check that your bulbs are not soft by giving them a gentle squeeze, and look out for any signs of mould.

There is a bulb for every situation and taste. If you don't want to take up planting space in a border or a vegetable bed, bulbs are perfect for containers, where they can be crammed in to provide a succession of spring flowers (*see below*). Some are fine in dappled shade (trillium, erythronium, narcissus and bluebell); others thrive in sunshine (tulips, allium and the delicate *Iris reticulata*, one of the first bulbs of the year). The majority of bulbs need good drainage to avoid rotting, so it is good practice to plant them on a layer of grit, if you can afford a small bag from the garden centre. However, it is not essential.

Many bulbs multiply from year to year, going from strength to strength, although the one notable exception is the tulip. The majority of them will disappoint in following years, and it is often best to dig them up once they have finished and buy new ones for next year.

Bulbs can be dotted around in awkward spots, such as under trees or in grass. In a mixed border, they can be planted in between herbaceous perennials that get going later in the year: as the bulbs are dying back, the foliage of the perennials takes over the space. This approach to the border has been dubbed 'succession planting', the idea being that one group of plants seamlessly takes over from another. Useful perennials to plant near bulbs include acanthus, Japanese anemones and many of the hundreds of hardy geraniums.

Spring bulbs can go in now, including those, such as alliums, that will be flowering into early summer. Tulips are accommodating, and you can get away with planting these as late as December. If you want snowdrops, it's best to wait until January and February: snowdrops (*Galanthus*) are best bought after they have flowered and planted 'in the green', which means as fully fledged plants (as opposed to bulbs), and when they have fully developed leaves.

Some ideas for bulbs

Bulbs in containers

We put our bulbs in large pots at the front of the school. Some daffodils will bloom as early as January, so if you want, you could try to stagger your display. Alternatively, you could go for a mix of bulbs: crocus, followed by daffodils, then tulips.

For a great show in a container using one sort of bulb, your container should have stone, gravel or bits of broken pot known as crocks in the bottom for drainage. Next, put in a layer of soil-based compost before placing your bulbs on top, almost touching, at the required depth (the rule of thumb is about three times the bulb's depth). Some gardeners then add horticultural grit to ensure good drainage, then more compost, but you can get away with compost if you don't have grit.

For a succession of daffodils, tulips and crocus in the same container, start with the daffs, about a bulb's width between them. The daffodils can go in quite deep: they will still find their way to the surface and it is better than going in too shallow – this is to risk them coming up 'blind' and not flowering. Next, fill in between

Autumn

project
Hyacinths for Christmas presents

Hyacinths in a border have never really done it for me. In a mixed border, there is something overly fussy about them, like a ball gown at a barn dance, while planted all together they remind me of municipal bedding. However, a few of them in a pot indoors, with their powerful scent and look-at-me blooms, is sensational – like experiencing an entirely different plant. The blue hyacinths are best for scent (try 'Blue Jacket'), while 'Amsterdam' is a stunning cerise colour. If you force them in the autumn, you can experience this in time for Christmas.

Forcing bulbs involves tricking the plants into thinking it is spring, usually by chilling them first, then bringing them into the warmth. You can buy your bulbs ready prepared or start the process off yourself by putting them in the fridge, wrapped in a paper bag, for at least four weeks. After chilling in the fridge, plant your bulbs in a mixture of horticultural grit and compost, with the tip just poking out of the surface. Bring them inside into the warmth and they should start to flower around six weeks later.

Note: When handling hyacinths, always wear gloves as the bulbs can irritate the skin.

the daffodils with grit or compost, with their tips showing. Now place the tulips in the gaps and repeat the process for the crocus.

Bulbs for naturalising in grass

Naturalising is where you plant bulbs to look as if they have arrived naturally in their setting. Think of swathes of spring bulbs in a seemingly carefree arrangement, in parks or on the lawn of a grand country house. Popular bulbs that might be used in a lawn or meadow situation include *Narcissus* 'Tête-à-Tête', *Crocus tomasinianus*, the tulip *Tulipa sprengerii* (very expensive bulbs but worth every penny), and a plant native to the North American prairie, camassia. If using bulbs in a lawn, it is important that the foliage is left to die back before mowing, as the leaves feed the bulbs for next year.

A word about alliums

If you are not familiar with the name, you will definitely recognise their appearance. Alliums, or ornamental onions, are typically purple or blue, lollipop-shaped plants with a globe of tiny flowers on top of a single, fat stem. They are lovely planted en masse or dotted around a border (I would use the same variety for the latter), and a useful bulb for a gardening club because they can be planted now, yet will perform in the summer term. The bog-standard allium – cheap as chips but still worth buying – is *A. hollandicum* 'Purple Sensation' (it grows to a height of around 1m). Smaller, yet with a globe that can be 20cm across and is made up of pronounced, star-like mini flowers is *A. cristophii*, also known as Star of Persia. This is lilac-coloured – as is another favourite, *A. giganteum*, which as the name suggests can grow to a height of 2m; the bulbs of the latter are expensive, but worth it and will bulk up year after year.

Like many bulbs, Mediterranean alliums want good drainage, so in a heavy soil it's worth putting grit underneath them when planting. They also want to be in full sun. Their uninteresting, strappy leaves are ugly when they die back, so gardeners often plant them among other perennials to conceal them.

If left to flower, the ornamental alliums' edible relative, the leek, makes a fabulous globe flower to rival any of its cousins. I have even seen trendy London florists selling these eye-catching vegetables for a fiver a stem. Suppliers include: Avon Bulbs (01460 242177; www.avonbulbs.co.uk).

PROS

- **Easy to grow outside or in containers.**
- **One investment means several years of blooms.**

CONS

- **Dying back foliage takes up a lot of space.**
- **Tall aliums prone to being blown over in windy spaces.**

Don't forget ...

- Check on the crops that stayed in the ground over summer.
- Earth up leeks and weed around them if necessary.

WEEK TWO

Sort out containers

One of the first jobs of the term is to sort out the bedraggled pots and hanging baskets that have spent the summer outside. For us, a few of the zinnias, gazanias and petunias were still clinging on, despite the holiday neglect, but we needed the pots for our spring bulbs (*see above*).

It is at this time of year that the newspaper supplements and gardening press advise you on how to pep up your containers. Sumptuous photographs tempt you with modish combinations of heathers, grasses and a sculptural evergreen or two (phormium, perhaps). But just look at the cost! Such containers could set you back £25. That's more than our budget for … well, we just wouldn't spend that on a pot.

Which varieties to grow?

Winter bedding is cheap, with a dozen baby plants costing between £3 and £4. Typical offerings include ornamental cabbages, kale, pansies and violas. Violas, though smaller flowered, tend to last longer than pansies, and so can be planted in the containers on top of bulbs. By the time the latter come through, the violas will have had it.

Note: at this time of year, plant bedding close together. You do not need to leave room for them to grow as you would do in spring and summer. These are not going to do much between now and the time you uproot them after Christmas.

PROS

- **Cheap bedding plants can be successfully grown in containers for winter colour.**

CONS

- **Not much to choose from out there, unless you're prepared to spend a lot of money.**
- **What you plant will remain static until spring.**

Don't forget ...

- Carry on cropping Swiss chard and perpetual spinach.
- Plant out or pot up strawberry runners.

did you know?

The aubergine is known to Americans and Australians as the eggplant because many of the earliest aubergines were white and looked like eggs. Two-thirds of the world's aubergines are grown in the US state of New Jersey.

WEEK THREE

Sow salad for winter

In September, it is getting late to sow salad leaves, but there are some things that you can get away with planting outdoors if the weather is OK, indoors if not. If you have a polytunnel or indoor space, or polythene cloches to go on the ground outdoors, this should be your preferred option. Your choice of what to grow is surprisingly rich for this time of year, providing you are not looking for fully grown plants but are prepared to harvest them as young, or cut-and-come-again leaves.

Many of the suggested salad leaves below have a strong flavour, and will be an acquired taste for most children. However, a mixed bag of salad is a nice thing to take home, especially in the closing months of the year.

One group of plants that likes the cooler, damp air of a British autumn is the Japanese greens, such as mizuna (tastes like a milder version of rocket) and red mustard (pungent to very hot, depending on how mature it is when you eat it). These are sown in late July and August outside, but can be sown in modules indoors during September, even October, and then transplanted outside.

Radicchio is the trendy, but sometimes overly bitter, leaf you'll find mixed into salads at this time of year. Treviso Precoce Mesola, however, is supposed to be less tough on the tastebuds.

Texsel, or Ethiopian, greens and land cress are both fast-growing, so suitable for this time of year. The former tastes like

Autumn

231

spinach and can be used the same way; the latter is like watercress, only with more coarse leaves. Rucola rocket is similarly fast-growing, while Russian kale can be harvested as a young leaf.

In our polytunnel, we planted winter purslane (aka claytonia or miner's lettuce). This germinated easily and, although it should survive outdoors, we kept it inside for a salady treat in early spring.

PROS

- **Salad in winter? Fabulous.**

CONS

- **Really best grown indoors.**
- **Nowhere near as prolific as spring- and summer-sown leaf.**

Don't forget ...

- If you have planted a meadow, it should be cut in late September/October.

WEEK FOUR

Sow broad beans

Broad beans were our first harvest at gardening club, plucked from a waterlogged square of clay we dared to call our garden. This says a lot for how easy they are to cultivate. Add to this the fact that they are delicious and no garden should be without them.

Which varieties to choose?

If you buy the right cultivar, you can sow broad beans in autumn for harvesting in the spring. With this timetable you risk losing them in a severe winter, but you also avoid the worst of the blackfly to which they are susceptible. If you lose your crop over winter, you can always plant some more in the early spring. Suitable cultivars for autumn planting include 'The Sutton' and 'Aquadulce Claudia'.

Pinch off the top of the plant when the first pods begin to form and start picking your beans when the pods are 6cm long. This should ensure tender young beans that maybe even the children will allow on their plates.

PROS
- **Really easy to grow.**
- **Something to plant in autumn when there is not much else that will grow.**
- **Provides an early spring crop.**

CONS

• **You might lose an autumn sowing to a severe winter.**

Don't forget ...

Cut back the stems of Jeruslaem artichokes (if they haven't fallen over already) and leave the tubers in the ground until needed.

did you know?

The bay leaf was held in high regard by the ancients. In classical times, the bay leaf was used to make the winner's crown in athletics games. Bay leaves were sacred to the ancient Greeks: in the temple at Delphi, which is dedicated to Apollo, the priestesses would eat whole bay leaves before delivering their prophecies. The Greeks also thought bay helped to protect against disease and used it as an antispetic. In Latin, bay is called *Laurus nobilis*, *laurus* meaning praise, *nobilis* meaning famous. From this is derived the term laureate, as in poet laureate.

WEEK FIVE

Sow sweet peas

If you have a sunny spot, grow sweet peas in the garden. They offer an irresistible combination of old-fashioned nostalgia with a beguiling simplicity of form. Then there's their knockout scent and the fact that they are so prolific that you can be generous with cutting them: take away one bloom and the plant will simply pump out more.

We had planted our first sweet peas in the spring term, and they seemed to take an age to germinate. This meant that they did not really hit their stride until the summer holidays, but we were lucky that the wet weather kept them going during the six-week break. By the beginning of autumn term they were still thriving, and well into October the children were cutting posies for teacher, Mum or Dad.

But planting sweet peas in the autumn term, and wintering them indoors, they get going that little bit earlier and should be flowering in June and July. You are in for the long haul, but it is worth it. If you get a wet summer holiday, which takes them through until September, then just see this as a bonus.

Sweet pea seeds are gnarled little pellets that belie the beauties they will turn into. Because of their rock-hard exterior, some growers advocate soaking the seed before planting, while others say you should nick them with a knife, the idea being that this helps them to germinate. Don't worry too much if you forget: you should still get your sweet pea seedlings.

235

Germination at this time of year, however, can be tricky if the seeds are not warm enough, so some gardeners prefer to start them off on a windowsill indoors. Otherwise, you run the risk of the seeds rotting. The moment they germinate, however, put them in a cold greenhouse, polytunnel or cold frame to prevent the seedlings growing too quickly and becoming leggy. If seedlings are looking thin and straggly, pinch out the tops to encourage them to bush out.

Sweet peas hate to have their roots disturbed when planted out, so are best sown individually or two at a time into decent sized pots (one litre) or root trainers (elongated plastic modules whose extra length should not check the growth of roots, and which open up at planting-out time to minimise disturbance to the young plant). Alternatively, a more environmentally friendly option is to use the cardboard centre of a toilet roll, as we do, standing them side by side in a seed tray before filling with compost. When it comes to planting, gently rip or slit open the cardboard before putting the seedling in the ground. Note: some advocates of this method say it is unnecessary to break open the cardboard, and that it will rot in the ground, but we have found that the decaying process takes too long and hinders the development of the young plant.

All being well, the sweet peas should be ready to plant out in late March or early April, depending on weather conditions and after a period of hardening off. This is the process of getting young plants used to life outdoors, typically by leaving them outside the polytunnel during the day and bringing them in for the night. If the weather is really mild, you could risk leaving them out, or get them into the ground straightaway. If it is really foul, wait until after the Easter break to do this.

Sweet peas need to be supported from the off, so canes should go into the ground before you plant them out to avoid damaging roots. You will not be over-ambitious using 2m supports, which should be pushed well into the soil so they do not, as has happened with us, end up toppling over. As they start growing outside, tie them in gently to the canes to encourage the tendrils to latch on to them.

As well as sowing your sweet peas at this time of year, you could also prepare the patch of ground that is to take them. Will they be planted in a wigwam or a straight line, with your canes laid out like an old-fashioned ridge tent? Let this dictate the area of earth you prepare.

Peas are very thirsty plants, so it is best to put them into earth that is rich in organic matter, which will better hold in moisture in the growing season. You could prepare the area with a rotted manure or garden compost. Traditionally, gardeners would dig a trench in the autumn, fill it with some of the contents of the compost heap – peelings, plant debris and ripped-up cardboard – then cover it over with earth. In the spring their peas would be planted in this space.

There is another advantage to starting sweet peas now, besides the fact that you will get them flowering in the summer term. If, for some reason, it all goes belly up, you still have next term to try again.

Which varieties to grow?

Up to you really; with sweet peas you really can throw good taste to the wind, and indulge in a mixed seed packet of clashing colours. There are, however, packs of single colour varieties, including Cathy Wright (white), Gwendoline (pink) and Windsor (maroon). My favourite are the pale blues and lilacs (try Albutt Blue or Honeymoon). Check out the specialists for a huge selection. Suppliers include Roger Parsons (01243 673770, rpsweetpeas.co.uk; Unwins (01480 443395, unwinsdirect.co.uk).

PROS

- **Flowers from June to October – the more you pick the more you get.**
- **Knockout scent.**
- **A stunning climber – all from a little seed. Sweet peas are often grown up a tepee with runner beans to attract pollinators to the latter. This is not needed with French beans, but the combination is fun and it can save on growing space.**

CONS

- **Can be prone to mould, but starting in pots usually gets round this.**

Don't forget ...

🌼 Rake any dead grass off the meadow.

WEEK SIX

Plant out garlic

Most strains of garlic need a cold period of 0–10°C for between 30 and 60 days; that is why it is planted in late autumn. When we got round to planting at gardening club it was late November. Ironically, after a freezing spell the week before, the weather was quite mild and dry. Of the seven children who turned up, no one was wearing a coat and one was only in a long-sleeved T-shirt. No one, of course, had brought their wellies.

Children don't generally like garlic, but it is easy to sneak into their food without them noticing. And they are not going to complain when they can plait the garlic bulbs after they have been harvested.

Our clay soil, prone to waterlogging, is not ideal for garlic, which prefers a well-drained soil. But the raised beds give us the necessary drainage. Alternatively, if you have a heavy soil and are worried the bulb will rot, plant the garlic on a layer of horticultural grit or sharp sand, or build up little ridges above the soil and plant into these.

Garlic should be grown in an open, sunny site. It is best not going into ground that has been recently manured. Too rich a soil and your garlic will put on top growth at the expense of the bulbs.

To plant garlic, break up a seed bulb into cloves, make a hole with a dibber or the handle of a trowel, then put a clove into the hole, pointed side up. Do not push the clove into the ground as this could damage it.

239

In a light soil, the cloves can be planted up to 10cm deep, but planting should be shallower in a heavy soil. However, they need at least 2.5cm of soil above them. Plant 10cm apart in rows with 30cm between them, or space them 18cm apart each way.

Then forget about them until the summer, when you will harvest them, minding that you keep the area weeded. You will know your bulbs are ready when the top growth starts to yellow and die back. Don't let the plants flower or their energy will go into the bloom and away from the bulb. Gently fork up the bulbs, taking care not to bruise them or they will rot in storage. Then, if you have fine

project

Making garlic plaits is a great thing to do with children. When bulbs are dry, tidy them up by pulling off loose stems and brushing off the soil, then dampen the stems and plait, three bulbs at a time or more, to be taken home or sold at the school gates.

For those who can't plait their own or their children's hair: lay three bulbs side by side with their stems intact. Gently tie the stems together next to the bulb with a bit of twine. Now, move the left hand stem over the centre stem, so that it is now in the middle. Next, move the right-hand stem over the centre stem, so that is now in the middle. Repeat, left, right, left, right, until the three stems make a plait.

weather, lay them out or hang them up in the sunshine to dry for about a week – if you don't trust the weather, you can do this in a well-ventilated indoor space such as a garage.

Which varieties to grow?

The first year you grow garlic, it is worth buying special seed bulbs, to make sure it is free from disease. You should also try to get an early variety to make sure you can crop it before the summer holidays: try Early Wight or for a purple variety Moldovan Wight. As seeds go, garlic is expensive, but you only have to buy them the first year. Thereafter, save a few of the fattest bulbs for breaking up and replanting the following autumn.

Suppliers include Edwin Tucker (01364 652233; www.edwin-tucker.com).

PROS

- **Easier to grow than it sounds, and a few bulbs go a long way.**
- **Stores well, and plaiting the bulbs makes a fun activity for the children.**

CONS

- **Many children associate garlic with spicy food, so don't like to eat it – one to sell at the school gates.**
- **Could rot in a heavy soil.**

Don't forget ...

- Harvest those Jerusalem artichokes, and if the school cook can't be persuaded to take them, sell them after school.

🌿 Next term's gardening club will come round really quickly. Don't forget to order next year's seed, to begin sowing in late February or March.

🌿 Did you plant any salad this autumn term? Can any be cut now before the holidays? If you are leaving anything in the polytunnel over Christmas – sweet peas, strawberries, cut-and-come-again salad – make a note to check on it early next year when it will need watering.

Autumn is also for ...

Onions

Government nutrition guidelines for lunches in primary schools state that each child should have at least two portions of fruit and vegetables per day. In our school kitchen – one of the few primary schools in the whole county that provides hot meals cooked on site – they struggle heroically to comply, and often augment these standards by sneaking more healthy stuff in by the back door. So, school mince (veggie and meat versions, both very popular) contains all manner of vegetables that, undisguised, would make some young children gag – chief among these is the onion.

Onions can be grown from seed, but are commonly available as small bulbs known as sets. These are much easier to grow and, if planted early in the autumn term, can be cropped in early summer. Make sure the sets are firm to the touch and don't plant any that are soft. Onions like a well-drained, sunny site and should not be planted on ground that is freshly manured or, like garlic, they will put on too much top growth at the expense of the bulbs.

How to sow

Plant in rows 30cm apart. Push the sets into the soil, about 10cm apart, with the pointed end on top and just visible. Onions have shallow roots, so weed carefully so as not to dislodge them. This also means that they can easily be uprooted by birds, and sometimes the action of frost. To keep birds away, tie lengths of cotton between stakes at either end of each row. Do not use netting, as some gardeners recommend, because birds can get tangled in it and die. I have a relative who is still traumatised by killing a thrush in this way some 20 years ago. If a growing bulb does become dislodged, dig a small hole and gently replant it.

Which varieties to grow?

When ordering sets, check they are right for your local climate. Popular cultivars for autumn sowing include Radar and, for a red onion, Electric. Onions can be harvested when you need them, and are ready to lift and store when the foliage dies back.

PROS

* Easily incorporated into school food.
* If sown as sets, they are less fiddly and more suitable for a school gardening club.
* Watering will be less of an issue with autumn-grown sets.

CONS

- **In very wet conditions, could be susceptible to rot – plant only in well-drained soil.**

Strawberries

Strawberries may be the quintessential summer fruit, with echoes of Wimbledon and cream teas, but autumn, when baby plants are available, is the time you should be thinking of growing them.

Before the gardening club, I had never really thought about growing strawberries. They seemed to be so much hassle compared with, say, raspberries, which will fruit year after year with little attention. I also think raspberries have a more predictable flavour, whereas with strawberries the flavour always seems to be a lottery.

Strawberries have to be cosseted, accessorised and defended like no other plant. Their many predators are enough to put you into a siege mentality. Just about every pest you can think of will, given the chance, have a go at the plants or their irresistible red fruits. From below, they are attacked by slugs. From above, they are dive-bombed by birds, while from the front and behind they have squirrels to contend with (whenever they get bored with raiding the bird feeder).

Strawberries are prone to mould if planted too close together, and mildew in dry weather. And if the plant makes it through to fruiting, they can be spoiled by mud or rot in the rain. Looking down the list of enemies and potential ailments, you would think there can't be many fruit or veg grown in this country that make such demands on your attention.

So why grow them in a gardening club with little time for fussing over such wimpish fruits and a high possibility of disappointment? My mind was made up when we found some strawberries growing happily in a forgotten corner. This part of the school grounds had been mostly left to its own devices, with a trim of a rosemary yearly and the occasional bit of weeding. During the past two summers, however, the strawberries had cropped fairly well – probably not to the standard or quantity of serious growers, but enough, for a few weeks, to distract the younger children whenever they got bored with what we were doing elsewhere. The fruit had not been protected by netting, as is recommended (though you risk killing a bird if it gets tangled up in it), and the plants had none of the paraphernalia you associate with them, such as special mats or straw to keep the fruit off the soil. They had been totally neglected, yet fruit had appeared for two seasons on the trot. The previous term, two six-year-old girls gathered enough in one day to fill a two-litre plant pot.

So if this small strawberry patch could produce fruit, maybe the gardening club should try cultivating some more. Strawberry plants are only good for three harvests before they should be discarded. We would have to hurry to get the next generation in place.

Strawberries need sunshine and well-drained soil. They are ideal planted along the side of a raised bed in an open site, which should drain well in winter (they don't like to be waterlogged) and, providing you have added compost or leaf mould, should retain some moisture in the ground in summer (strawberries don't like to get too dry, so might need watering in hotter months). Strawberries don't want the soil to be too nutrient-rich, as this will mean more leaf growth at the expense of fruit. And they need a winter chill to make sure they flower the following year. The plants should be put in with their crowns (the central bit where the stems come up) just above soil level. Space them about 50cm apart.

Alternatively, you can grow them in containers, the larger the better so that they do not dry out, and where they will be away from predators on the ground. We planted our strawberries in 25cm pots and a large hanging basket, to spend the winter in the polytunnel, before planting them outdoors in early spring. They can go straight in the ground at the end of summer, but we had left it rather late. Our strawberries were in potting compost, so would not need feeding over spring and into summer, but they would need to be fed after cropping the following year.

It is best to buy your strawberries from a reputable supplier or garden centre, where they will be certified disease-free. But once you have an established bed, more plants are easily propagated. Strawberries reproduce by sending out stems, or stolons, from the main plant, which then root, forming baby plants, or runners, at their ends. When runners begin to form, they should be removed so as not to weaken the main plant, but you can leave on one or two to be transplanted into pots for the next generation of plants.

Top Tip

Strawberry plants are only good for three harvests before they should be discarded.

Which varieties to grow?

Popular varieties that will crop before the end of the summer term include Honeoye and Pegasus, the latter having a reputation for good resistance to disease. Suppliers include Welsh Fruit Stocks (01497 851209; www.welshfruitstocks.co.uk) and the Organic Gardening Catalogue (0845 130 1304; www.organiccatalogue.com).

Seed saving works

I am a late convert to saving seed, partly because I have always thought there is little point in it when you can pick up a whole packet so cheaply, and partly because, like making perfectly raised scones, I suspected it was a lot more difficult than its advocates claimed it to be. Exceptions are the self-seeding beasts of the flower bed such as forget-me-not, calendula and certain poppies – not only is it hard for these to fail, but if not kept in check they can become a nuisance.

However, I decided to try it with *Verbena bonariensis*, an undemanding perennial with purple clusters of tiny flowers on top of tall, thin stems.

I love this plant for its long season and the fact that despite its size you can slot it in anywhere in the garden. At the back of the border you still catch sight of its flowerheads, popping up between clumps of large herbaceous plants and shrubs; at the front, its stems become invisible and you look through them to what is planted behind. Insects love this plant, too,

Autumn

247

and in early autumn when many perennials are looking rough or have given up completely, it is still going strong.

Growing it from seed is, I find, a doddle. So easy that within a season, I have more plants than I would ever need, all of them as robust as the ones selling at the garden centre for £6 a pot. Never again will I knock seed saving.

Now, experienced gardeners reading this might sneer and say that *Verbena bonariensis* needs no helping hand to multiply. Leave it be and it will seed freely all over the garden. But this approach is flawed – it relies on the existence of undisturbed areas of land where the seedlings can get a start. In any garden under intense cultivation, where hoeing is used to keep down weeds and to disturb pests such as slugs, you are going to be less successful with self-seeders.

Collecting and saving seed is a great activity for children. In the summer, you can gather the heads of early flowering annuals and perennials such as Welsh poppy and aquilegia. In early autumn, we gathered ripe bean pods, now too mature and tough to eat, emptied their seeds and put them in an envelope to plant the following spring. Tagetes and rudbeckia got a similar treatment, too.

The key to seed saving is to emulate nature as far as possible. Collect your seeds just before the plant is about to disperse them. This doesn't involve hanging around decaying plants waiting for the seed heads to pop, but keep your eyes open. As the leaves of the plant begins to dry up, it means the seeds will be ripening, so you should place a paper bag over the top of a flower head, sever the stem and invert the whole thing.

Next, tie the bag at the top before putting it somewhere to dry – hung from the roof of a classroom with good ventilation, for example. A paper bag is important: the seeds might rot in a plastic one.

Your seeds could then go straight in the ground (as nature intended), but that would leave them prone to the hoe (not as nature intended), pest attacks, competition from other plants and, in the case of autumn-sown seeds, extremes of weather. Why make it hard for yourself, and disappointing for children, should the seeds fail to germinate? Better, I reckon, to plant them straightaway in pots and put them under cover, to give them a head start, or save them and plant them in the spring.

There is nothing quite like raising a plant yourself – the important thing is to try first with easier plants, and experiment with others if this is a success. At the gardening club we have been successful with broad beans and have calendula seeds and French beans ready to put in for next year. I'll be saving more difficult plants for another day. Six easy plants from which to collect seed are aquilegia, Welsh poppy, nasturtium, Opium poppy, broad beans and sweet peas.

Autumn

Planting perennials

Technically, a perennial is any plant that carries on year after year, which would include trees and shrubs, but generally when a gardener refers to a perennial, they mean those of the herbaceous kind. So, if you have heard someone refer to a herbaceous border, it means one primarily composed of these plants, and one that is typical of gardens both grand and more modest around the country. These borders will probably also have spring bulbs and shrubs dotted around them, so are more correctly referred to as mixed borders.

Buying perennials in pots can soon get expensive, but looked at as a one-off investment, they are remarkably good value. Herbaceous perennials come back year after year, dying back in winter and pushing out new shoots in the spring. A single spending spree and a few hours planting them can turn one year's sad little corner of the garden into next season's stunner.

Certain perennials can be divided year after year, so getting more plants from your initial investment. It might seem counter-intuitive to buy them at this time of year, when many of them are past their best, but if you get them in the ground now, they have time to get established before next year's growing season.

Perennials in pots can be sourced, and planted, all year round, except in extreme weather when it's too hot, cold or dry. Planting them in the autumn, however, means you don't have to worry about watering them while they are dormant, whereas spring- or summer-planted perennials will need more attention and watering.

When planting perennials – or indeed any plant from a pot – first soak it in a bucket of water. If it is pot-bound (the roots exposed in a tangle where the compost meets the pot) gently tease out the roots at the edges. This will encourage them to grow into the soil.

The only problem with buying perennials at this time of year can be sourcing them from mainstream garden centres, who only want to display plants that are in their prime, rather than those that gave their best earlier in the year and are now biding their time until they die off for winter. A good nursery, however, will know that true gardeners make allowances for such things, and are not expecting the horticultural equivalent of a sweet shop. So find a local nursery with a good reputation or buy mail order: you'll get help with both in the Royal Horticultural Society's Plantfinder directory, or online at www.rhs.org.uk.

Six easy perennials

All the plants listed below have a long season, need little attention and should give some interest on one or both sides of the summer holidays. Plant in a well-drained soil that has been prepared with plenty of organic matter.

Acanthus spinosus, or bear's breeches: A reliable architectural plant with large, divided leaves and a statuesque flower spike that can reach 1.5m. You can plant spring bulbs around its base and the large leaves, about 40cm long, that emerge later in the spring will cover up the dying foliage of the bulbs. Acanthus is subtle on colour (with spiky bracts of purple and white on the stem) but big on stature: a real eye-catcher, happy in sunshine or partial shade.

Aster: Many forms of the traditional Michaelmas daisy are prone to powdery mildew at the end of summer, to such an extent that many gardeners don't bother with asters any more. Aster Little Carlow, however, is an exception. Its smallish violet-blue flowers with yellow centres appear mid-summer, but will still be going strong when school reconvenes in September. Easy to propagate by dividing in spring. Prefers sun and grows to a height of about 90cm.

Geranium: There are hundreds of hardy geraniums, or cranesbills, on the market, and some of them flower for months on end. Their palmate leaves tend to form clumps, some of a more straggly habit than others, but their appeal is in their pretty, often simple, saucer-shaped flowers. *Geranium endressii* is pink with a very long season, 'Rozanne' and 'Brookside' are blue-flowered, while 'Ann Folkhard', which likes to send out its dainty flowers on long, exploring stems and pop up through other plants, has magenta blooms with a black centre.

After their first flush in midsummer, geraniums can be cut back to the soil, given a dousing of water, and they will return with fresh new growth, and often more flowers, later in the summer.

Japanese anemone: I would always go for one of the single-flowered varieties of this lovely plant, many of which get going in early summer and are still flowering in October. *Anemone x hybrida* 'Honorine Jobert' has simple white flowers with a yellow centre that rise on sturdy stems up to 1.5m high. 'Honorine Jobert' is the most common one you will come across at a garden centre, often more conveniently labelled Japanese anemone. These plants can take a while to settle in, not performing well in their first season in the ground, but after that they bulk up and you should have no problems with them. They are happy in sun or shade and are another useful plant around which to put spring bulbs – their clump-forming foliage does not get going until later in the spring, at which time it will cover up the mess of dying bulb leaves around it. My favourite Japanese anemones, however, are the single pink varieties: try *Anemone x hybrida* 'Elegans' and *A. hupehensis.*

Knautia macedonica: Deep magenta pincushion flowers on stems that project out from a leafy clump. After the first flowers start to die back in summer, you can cut it back with shears, douse in a bucket of water, and it will come back again, flowering well into the autumn. A cottage garden favourite, it likes full sun and grows to a height of about 70cm.

Sedum spectabile: Another late summer-autumn flowerer and confirmed favourite for butterflies. I have seen clouds of these insects hovering around the tiny blooms that make up pink, flat flower heads on stems about 40cm high. When these die off in late autumn, they turn a dried russet colour and will hang on into winter before eventually collapsing. Sedums insist on good drainage, but are generally undemanding. Easily propagated by division in the spring.

Feeding the birds

An important job over autumn and winter is keeping the birds fed, when sources of food are few and far between. Can you hang up bird feeders around the school, or perhaps invest in a bird table?

More important than food is making sure the birds have access to water in freezing weather.

What should they be washing down with that water? Bread is of little nutritional use to birds, so don't overdo it with the crusts and crumbs. Good things to feed them include cooked, unsalted rice, porridge oats, sultanas, currants, raisins, cheese, pastry and cold potatoes. They'll repay your kindness in spring and summer, helping to keep slugs, snails and aphids at bay. In the garden, as in many walks of life, a little understanding goes a long way.

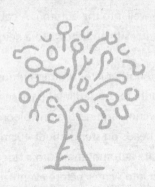

aPPendices

Glossary

Allium: Any member of the allium genus of plants, which includes onions, shallots, leeks, chives and garlic.

Annual: A plant whose life cycle – from seed germination to the death of the plant – only lasts one year.

Biennial: A plant that grows over two seasons, usually flowering and/or fruiting in the second before dying off.

Biodiversity: The abundance and range of animals, plants, fungi and micro-organisms present in any environment, as fostered by organic gardening.

Biological control: Using another creature to attack a pest infestation, such as introducing ladybird larvae to feast on aphid-covered leaves.

Bolting: A term used to describe a vegetable crop that has become worthless because it has started to flower and set seed. Can be a problem with salad crops as warm weather causes some varieties to flower.

Brassica: Any member of the brassica genus of plants, such as cabbage, rocket, cress, cauliflower, Brussels sprouts and kale.

Chitting: Encouraging seed potatoes to sprout before planting them in the ground. Achieved by placing in a light, cool place.

Cloche: A clear glass or plastic cover, traditionally bell-shaped, used to cover individual plants or groups of plants to protect them from frosts or temperature extremes.

Cold frame: A wooden or aluminium-framed structure with a hinged glass or clear plastic lid that is used to protect plants from extremes of weather. *See Hardening off.*

Comfrey tea: Comfrey contains high levels of nitrogen, so a solution of comfrey leaves, having sat for some weeks in water, works as an organic liquid feed when watered on plants. Nettles can be used as an alternative to comfrey.

Companion planting: A planting scheme where plants that provide some benefit to a crop are grown close to that crop. For instance, the strong odours of onion, chive and garlic plants are believed to mask the smell of carrots, thereby throwing the destructive carrot fly off the scent.

Crop rotation: A growing regime that groups plants into several categories according to their needs; usual groupings are the potato family, legumes, brassicas and roots. In the first year, each group is grown on a particular area of the allotment; the following year the beds are 'rotated' in a specific order so that the plants always receive the best possible soil conditions and no group grows on the same soil in consecutive years.

Crown: The part of a plant where the stems meet the roots; usually positioned at soil level when planting.

Cultivar: Shorthand for cultivated variety: a strain of plant that has been developed by gardeners through selective breeding.

Cut-and-come-again: A leafy salad crop – lettuce, corn salad, Chinese greens, and so on – that is picked as individual leaves when the plant is still young, and expected to continue to grow, providing a continuous harvest.

Damping off: A fungal disease that kills seedlings, making them collapse from the stem. Prevalent in damp conditions.

Deadheading: Removing the flower heads from plants as they fade in order to prolong the flowering period.

Dibber: A pointed stick, usually wooden, used to make holes in the earth for sowing seeds and planting bulbs or seedlings.

Double digging: A method of preparing a bed for planting, generally used for compacted or poorly drained soil, in which sections of soil are dug into trenches and the bottom of the trench is broken up with a fork.

Drill: A shallow groove made in the soil for sowing seed.

Earthing up: Piling up earth around the base and stem of a plant. Mostly used to prevent light from reaching potato tubers and celery stems and to deter weeds.

Fertiliser: Any material added to soil to provide varying amounts of soluble nitrogen, phosphorus and potassium, all of which are nutrients that help plants to grow. Includes manure, comfrey tea and commercially available brands.

Fleece: A thin, white, lightweight material that protects plants from harsh weather while allowing light to reach them, aand keeps out pests. Also known as horticultural fleece.

Forcing: Putting a plant – usually rhubarb or seakale – into the dark, usually by means of a bucket or a tall lidded terracotta pot specially designed for the purpose, in December or January so that it produces delicate, tasty shoots.

Green manure: A crop, such as field beans or rye grass, that is grown to improve the quality and fertility of the soil rather than for eating. Often left to stand over the winter and dug into the ground in the spring. Also known as cover crops or living mulches.

Half-hardy: Plants that can be grown outdoors after the risk of frost has passed

Hardening off: The process of gradually exposing seedlings grown indoors or in a greenhouse to the harsher conditions of the outside in preparation for planting them out on the plot.

Hardy: Any plant that can survive without cover or other protection throughout the year, including the winter.

Heritage vegetable: A variety of plant that is pollinated by natural means (the wind, insects, birds and so on) and was introduced before 1951 but has ceased to be grown commercially because it doesn't conform to the requirements of industrial-scale agriculture. Heritage vegetables are prized by some gardeners for their unique qualities, history and flavour. Also known as an heirloom vegetable.

Hot bed: A cold frame that is positioned over a layer of fresh manure which, as it breaks down, releases heat to warm the structure. Used as a mini-greenhouse to raise crops when temperatures outdoors are too low.

Humus: The organic material contained within soil, created when organisms such as worms and bacteria break down dead plant matter.

Leaf mould: Decomposed leaves that can be used as a medium for seed sowing and as a way of adding humus to soil.

Legume: Any member of the Leguminosae (also known as Fabaceae) family, especially peas and beans. Includes runner beans, fenugreek, broad beans and lupins.

Lime: A calcium compound spread on to soil as a dressing to raise its pH (make it less acidic and more alkaline).

Loam: A rich soil ideal for cultivating fruit and vegetables. Contains equal quantities of sand, clay and silt and is full of organic material.

Mulch: Material that is layered thickly on the surface of the soil to retain water, suppress weeds and prevent the leaching of nutrients. Many different materials can be used for mulch, including black plastic sheeting, wads of newspaper, cardboard and grass cuttings.

Nematode: A family of tiny parasitic worms. Some nematodes, such as Phasmarhabditis hermaphrodita, can be used to control pests such as slugs. Others can damage plants, for example eelworms, which eat roots and potato tubers.

Nitrogen fixer: Plants from the legume family that can help to enrich the soil with nitrogen. Bacteria that live in the plants' roots take nitrogen from the air and convert it into a form that plants can use as an essential soil nutrient. The nitrogen is then stored in the plants until they are incorporated into the soil and decompose, gradually releasing the nitrogen into the soil where it can once more be taken up by subsequent crops. Many green manures are also nitrogen fixers.

Nodule: A growth on the roots of certain plants that hosts bacteria which take nitrogen from the air and store it.

Nutrient: Mineral substance absorbed by the roots of plants. The most important nutrient is nitrogen, followed by phosphorus and potash (potassium). Nutrients are not always beneficial and problems can arise if concentrations are too high. Excess nitrogen can result in too leafy growth and delay flowering and fruiting.

Offset: A young plant that grows out from the body of a mature plant and develops its own root system. It can be removed and transplanted to create a second plant.

Organic gardening: Working with nature to boost the productivity and natural health of the soil in order to grow plants without the use of synthetic chemicals.

Organic matter: Anything that rots down easily such as manure, compost or vegetable waste.

Overwintering: Planting specially prepared seeds or sets in the late summer or autumn which will start growing, survive the winter and supply you with an early spring harvest. Specially 'overwintered' or 'overwintering' varieties of peas, garlic, broad beans, lettuce and onions are some of the most popular crops for overwintering.

Perennial: A plant that will survive for several years.

Perlite: A lightweight, white, granular substance used in potting-compost mixes because it holds water and helps aerate the soil.

Pinch out: To remove a plant's shoots in order to check its growth or train it in a certain way.

Plug plants: Young plants that are too old to be classed as seedlings but are not yet fully grown. Usually sold in module trays and ready to plant out immediately.

Pollination: The transfer of pollen – either by wind, insects, birds or human hand – between the sexual organs of plants as a precursor to the fertilisation of seed. Cross-pollination occurs when the transfer is between two different plants; self-pollination is when the pollen is moved either between two different flowers on the same plant, or between the sexual organs of a single flower.

Prick out: To transplant young seedlings from a seed tray or pot into individual pots.

Propagating: Growing new plants by using various techniques, such as taking cuttings, sowing seeds or removing offsets.

Pruning: Removing stems from a plant in a bid to make it more productive. Commonly used on soft fruit such as raspberries and blackcurrants.

Raised bed: A growing bed edged with wood, plastic or some other material and filled with extra soil to lift it above the level of the surrounding paths. Favoured by many vegetable growers as a less labour-intensive way of growing.

Rust: A fungal disease that can affect broad beans, onions, leeks and garlic. The symptoms are rusty red pustules on the leaves and stems in the summer months.

Seed potatoes: Specially-treated potato tubers that are bought by growers and prepared for planting by being sprouted (or chitted as it's also known). When placed in the ground the sprouts will grow upwards and each tuber will produce a single potato plant, which can yield dozens of potatoes.

Sets: Small, specially prepared bulbs of either onions or shallots that can be planted instead of sowing seed and will grow into full-sized bulbs.

Soil improver: Any organic material added to the soil to improve its fertility and general condition, including leaf mould, mushroom compost and rotted manure.

Soil pH: A measure of how acid or alkaline a patch of soil is. The pH scale goes from 0 to 14: soil with pH 7 is neutral, pH 0 to 7 is increasingly acidic, and pH 7 to 14 is increasingly alkaline. Most soil in the UK falls between 4 and 9. Soil pH can dictate what plants you can grow, as some won't thrive in acid or alkaline conditions.

Station sowing: Sowing seeds in their final growing position, far enough apart that little or no thinning is required. Often used for larger seeds such as squash and beans, where two seeds are planted together to ensure that at least one seed germinates in each spot – if two seedlings grow, the weaker one is removed.

Succession planting or sowing: A little and often approach to sowing seeds, resulting in a crop that matures over a number of weeks or months rather than all at once.

Tilth: Soil that has been prepared for growing. It should be crumbly and fine, free from large stones and with plenty of organic material.

Trench composting: A shortcut way of composting that entails burying green and kitchen waste in the ground and covering with soil several months before the start of the growing season. Particularly useful when preparing the ground for growing crops that thrive on rich soil, such as pumpkins, courgettes and beans.

Truss: A stalk that ends in a cluster of flowers or fruit. Most often used to describe the flowering stems of tomato plants.

Vermiculite: A lightweight, flaky mineral used in potting-compost mixes for its water retention and aerating qualities.

Wormcasts: Piles of fine, humus-rich soil that are excreted by worms. Can be harvested from wormeries or bought and applied to your plot as a soil improver.

Wormery: A bin containing worms that's used as a faster, more efficient way to compost kitchen waste and generate organic fertiliser.

RESOURCES

Support and Information

BBC Gardening. Information galore on many aspects of gardening, both in-depth or beginners' stuff. Also has a dedicated section to gardening with children. www.bbc.co.uk/gardening

British Potato Council Potatoes for Schools. Free spuds. Online activities for children and information for teachers. www.potatoesforschools.org.uk

Edible Playground. A new scheme supporting schools across the country with growing tips and, in a limited number of cases, seeds and equipment, too. www.edibleplayground.co.uk

Federation of City Farms and Community Gardens. Works primarily in urban areas advising on community projects and, in some cases, school farms. Also, plenty of ideas for places to visit. www.farmgarden.org.uk

Food for Life Partnership. A group of organisations, including the Soil Association and Health Care Trust, which have got together to encourage healthy eating in schools. Possible support for growing in your school. www.foodforlife.org.uk

Garden Organic for Schools. Part of the venerable Garden Organic website. In-depth information for children and teachers, linking activities, where appropriate, to the National Curriculum www.gardenorganic.org.uk/schools_organic_network

Growing Schools. A government scheme to get children of all ages to use and appreciate the outdoors more. It includes suggestions for possible funding and case studies on individual schools. Get Your Hands Dirty (www.teachernet.gov.uk/growingschools/resources/ teachingresources/detail.cfm?id=298) has a wealth of practical information on starting and running a school garden. www.teachernet.gov.uk/growingschools

Herb Society. The website includes a school section with fact sheets, activities and information on what other schools are doing. www.herbsociety.org.uk/schools

Learning Through Landscapes. Practical help on developing your school grounds. www.ltl.org.uk

Little Rotters. Loads of advice about composting. Aimed specifically at primary schools, but just as useful for beginners. www.littlerotters.org.uk

Royal Horticultural Society. This exhaustive website from the gardening establishment is an essential tool for every gardener, young and old. In 2007, it launched its campaign for school gardening. Sign up for free seeds and a goody bag. www.rhs.org.uk/schoolgardening

Seedy Sunday. An annual event for swapping unusual and heritage seeds. The useful little website has information on other similar schemes around the country. www.seedysunday.org

Seed, plants and equipment

Chiltern Seeds, 01229 581137, www.chilternseeds.co.uk

Dobies Seeds, 0844 701 7625, www.dobies.co.uk

DT Brown, 0845 166 2275, www.dtbrownseeds.co.uk

Edulis, 01635 578113, www.edulis.co.uk

Edwin Tucker, 01364 652233, www.edwintucker.com

Garden Organic Heritage Seed Library, 02476 303517,
    www.gardenorganic.co.uk

Green Gardener, 01603 715096, www.greengardener.co.uk

Jekka's Herb Farm, 01454 418878, www.jekkasherbfarm.com

Mr Fothergills, 0845 371 0518, www.mr-fothergills.co.uk

Rocket Gardens, 0845 603 3684, www.rocketgardens.co.uk

Seeds of Italy, 020 8427 5020, www.seedsofitaly.co.uk

Suttons, 0844 922 2899, www.suttons.co.uk

Tamar Organics, 01579 371087, www.tamarorganics.co.uk

The Organic Gardening Catalogue, 01932 253666,
    www.organiccatalog.com

The Real Seed Catalogue, 01239 821107, www.realseeds.co.uk

Thomas Etty, 01460 57934, www.thomasetty.co.uk

Thompson & Morgan, 0844 248 5383, www.thompson-morgan.com

W Robinson & Son, 01524 791210, www.mammothonion.co.uk

Wiggly Wigglers, 01981 500391, www.wigglywigglers.co.uk

Selected bibliography

Encyclopedia of Organic Gardening, edited by Pauline Pears
    (Dorling Kindersley)

Garden Flowers, by Christopher Lloyd (Cassell)

Garden Natural History, by Stefan Buczacki (Collins)

Grow Your Own Veg, by Carol Klein (Mitchell Beazley)

Grow Your Own Vegetables, by Joy Larkcom (Frances Lincoln)

Meadows, by Christopher Lloyd (Cassell)

New Gardening, by Matthew Wilson (Mitchell Beazley)

Organic Bible, by Bob Flowerdew (Kyle Cathie)

Organic Gardening the Natural No Dig Way, by Charles Dowding
    (Green Books)

Pests, Diseases and Disorders of Garden Plants, by Stefan Buczacki and
    Keith Harris (Collins)

Sticky Wicket, by Pam Lewis (Frances Lincoln)

Succession Planting for Adventurous Gardeners, by Christopher Lloyd
    (BBC Books)

The Allotment Handbook, by Caroline Foley (New Holland)

The Allotment Keeper's Handbook, by Jane Perrone (Atlantic)

The Curious Gardener's Almanac, by Niall Edworthy (Eden Project Books)

The First Time Naturalist, by Nick Baker (Collins)

The Great Vegetable Plot, by Sarah Raven (BBC Books)

The Greenhouse Gardener, by Anne Swithinbank (Frances Lincoln)

The Organic Garden, by Allan Shepherd (Collins)

Vegetables, Herbs and Fruit, by Matthew Biggs, Jekka McVicar and
    Bob Flowerdew (Firefly)

How to get vegetables to crop in term time

Vegetable	When to sow/plant	Plant out
Beetroot	Late February-March indoors	Mid April when first true leaves appear
Broad bean	Autumn or early spring outdoors	
Carrot	Early March indoors, late March outdoors	When seedlings are 2.5cm high
Courgette	Mid April indoors	After all risk of frost, from mid-May onwards
French bean	Mid April indoors	After all risk of frost, from mid-May onwards
Garlic	Late autumn outdoors	
Jerusalem artichoke	February onwards outdoors	
Leaf beet	April outdoors	
Leek	March indoors	Seed trays can go outside in May. Transplant when the width of a pencil
Microgreens	Any time indoors	
Onion sets	October outdoors	
Peas (mangetout)	From March outdoors	
Potato	Late March outdoors	
Pumpkin	Mid-April indoors	Mid-May after the frosts
Salad leaf including rocket & Japanese greens	March-June indoors and outdoors, also September indoors	
Tomato	Late February/early March indoors	

Easy rating	Notes
xxx	Bolt-resistant varieties needed for indoor planting
xxx	Spring sowing is more likely to have a blackfly problem in the summer
x	Heavy soil and carrot root fly are big problems
xx	To guarantee a crop before the end of term, try growing on in containers indoors
xx	A favourite of slugs and snails
xxx	Soil must be well draining
xxx	Good for breaking in new soil
xxx	Unlikely to be fully mature before the summer holidays. Harvest as cut-and-come again or young leaves
xxx	Occupies land for a long time
xxx	Perfect if you have no outside space
xx	Need well-drained soil. Protect from birds
xx	Essential that plants are given support
xxx	Essential that you 'earth-up' plants as they grow
xx	A plant really for the children to take home, though you could risk some in the ground over the summer holiday
xx	Indoor sowings mean plants more likely to survive pests
x	Best to grow tomatoes indoors or for the children to take young plants home

Easy rating XXX=Very easy XX=Easy X=Could need some TLC

Index

Endnote

During the writing of this book, the gardening club had become involved in a new initiative called Edible Playgrounds (www.edibleplaygrounds.co.uk), to encourage the growing of food in schools.

One way of promoting the scheme was a garden at the Chelsea Flower Show, and our gardening club was asked if some of the children would 'open' it to the press.

Of course, we were honoured. So, in May 2008, a small group of us travelled to London for the horticultural event of the year. We were an incongruous sight – Chelsea does not normally permit children on to its hallowed ground – and some eyebrows were raised among the colonels in blazers and ladies in silly hats. But the papers, radio and television loved it and spent some time interviewing the students.

While all this was going on, celebrity gardener Joe Swift dropped in for a photo call. I pointed out that the children had grown the beetroot in the display, it's crimson leaves in pride of place among other veg supplied by the nation's top growers. 'Very nice,' said Joe; 'just don't ask me to eat it.'

The best, however, was yet to come. Back in Dorset the next day, we heard the Edible Playground had not only been awarded a coveted gold medal, but had won Best Courtyard Garden at the show. This was a huge achievement for the garden's designer Nick Williams-Ellis and a great boost to the scheme. And, playing a small but significant part in this success, was some beetroot grown by a group of kids.